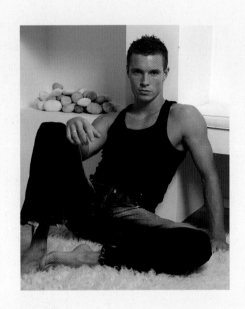

Ultimate
GAY SEX

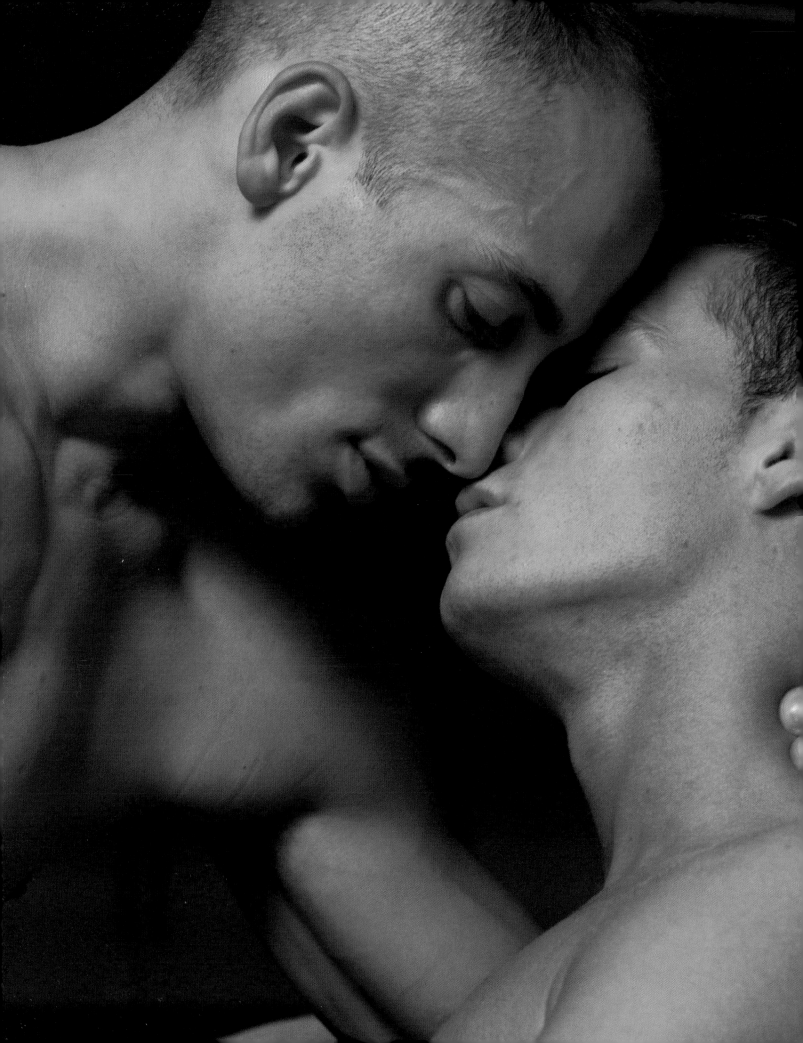

Ultimate
GAY SEX

Michael Thomas Ford

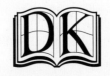

DK Publishing, Inc.

LONDON, NEW YORK, MUNICH,
MELBOURNE, DELHI

Senior Editor Jennifer Williams
Senior Art Editor Susan St. Louis
Editorial Consultant Peter Jones
Art Director Dirk Kaufman
DTP Designer Milos Orlovic
Production Chris Avgherinos, Heather Hughes
Picture Research Carolyn Clerkin, Chrissy McIntyre
Picture Librarians Claire Bowers, Romaine Werblow
Photography Justin Slide
Project Director Sharon Lucas
Creative Director Tina Vaughan
Publisher Chuck Lang

Produced for DK Publishing, Inc. by

studio cactus ltd

13 SOUTHGATE STREET WINCHESTER HAMPSHIRE SO23 9DZ UK
TEL 00 44 1962 878600 **FAX** 00 44 1962 859278
E-MAIL MAIL@STUDIOCACTUS.CO.UK **WEBSITE** WWW.STUDIOCACTUS.CO.UK

Senior Editor Aaron Brown
Senior Art Editor Dawn Terrey
Designers Sharon Rudd, Laura Watson
Creative Director Amanda Lunn
Editorial Director Damien Moore

First American Edition, 2004
04 05 06 07 08 10 9 8 7 6 5 4 3 2 1

Published in the United States by
DK Publishing, Inc.
375 Hudson Street
New York, New York 10014

Published in Great Britain in 2004 by
Dorling Kindersley Limited
80 Strand, London, WC2R 0RL

DK Publishing, Inc. offers special discounts for bulk purchases for sales
promotions or premiums. Specific, large-quantity needs can be met
with special editions, including personalized covers, excerpts of existing
guides, and corporate imprints.
For more information, contact: Special Markets Department,
DK Publishing, Inc., 375 Hudson Street, New York, New York 10014
Fax 212-689-5254.

Cataloging-in-Publication data is available from the Library of Congress
US ISBN 0-7894-9697-6

Cataloging-in-Publication data is available from the British Library
UK ISBN 1-4053-0328-X

Color reproduction by GRB Editrice s.r.l., Italy
Printed and bound in Italy by LEGO

See our complete product line at
www.dk.com

First printing, May 2004

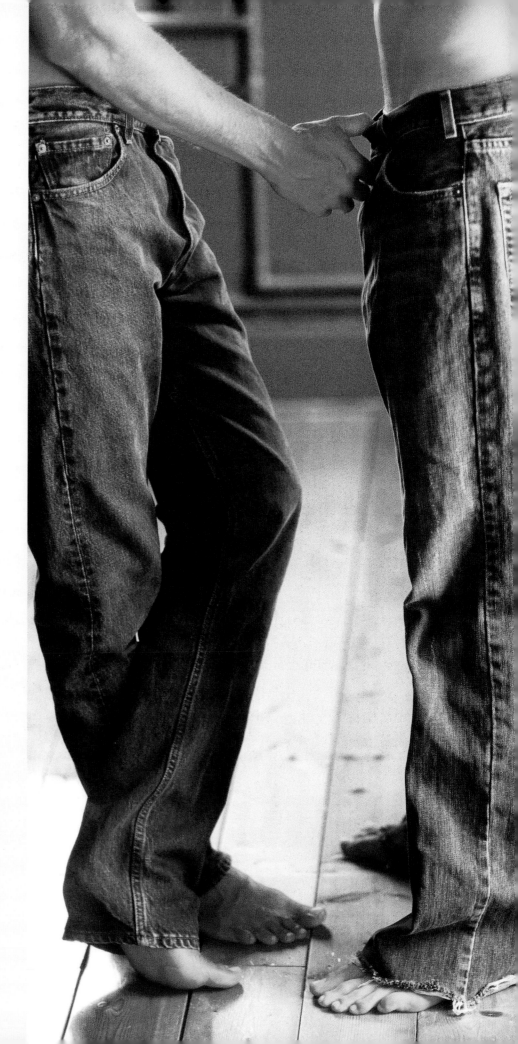

Contents

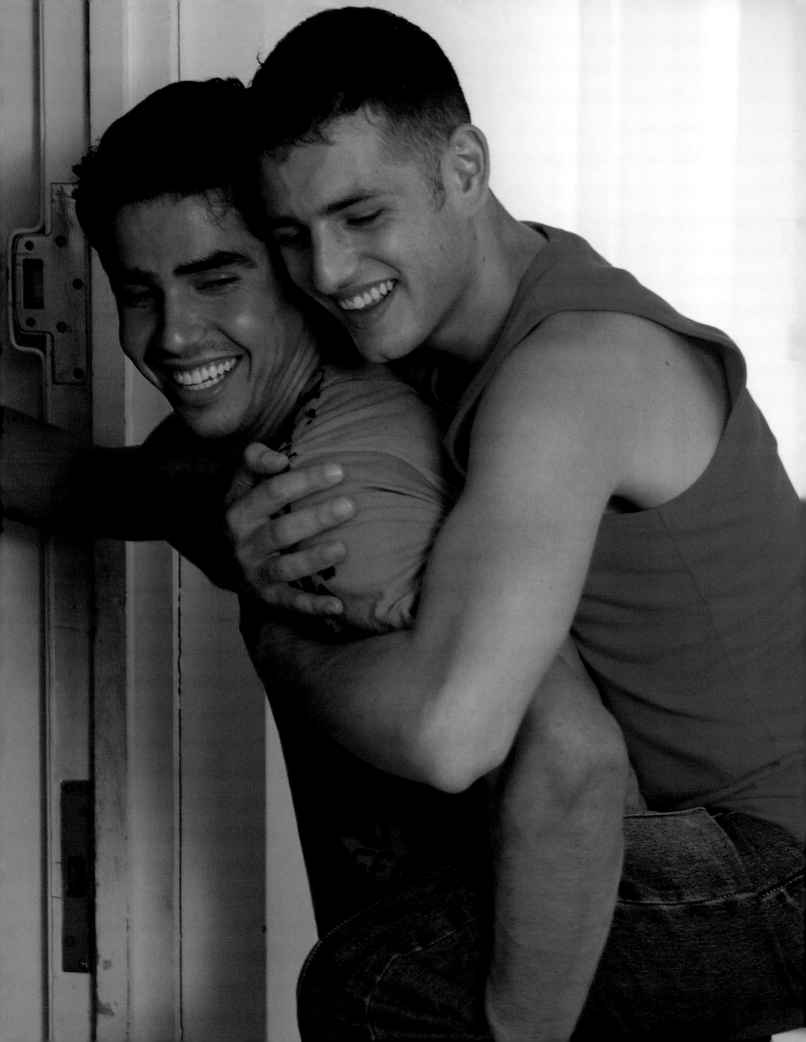

Introduction

They say men think about sex something like once every six minutes. You'd think after all that thinking we'd all be experts at actually *having* sex. Sadly, this is not the case. Often when we try to bring the fantasies in our heads to life in the bedroom, many of us are less than proficient at it, and some of us are downright clumsy.

But there is hope. The truth is, sex isn't all that complicated. Yes, there are some basic maneuvers you need to master before you can really be great at it, but basically it's about as difficult as riding a bike or learning how to get a barbeque going. You just have to practice it a few times, or maybe a lot of times. But at some point a little light goes on in your head and a voice says, "Ah-ha! So *that's* where that goes and *that's* what that does."

Okay, so it's slightly more complicated than that. But not by very much. Here's a secret—good sex is mostly in your head, not in your pants. We tend to forget this. Great sex has to start in the imagination. It has to be something that grows out of knowing what turns us, and our partners on, otherwise it's just a couple of body parts smacking together while we huff and puff.

The purpose of this book is to get you thinking about sex. Yes, we'll talk about some techniques you can try, and we'll discuss a lot of sex-related issues that you should know about. But really what I want is for you to start thinking about what sex means to you. Why do you enjoy it? What does it do for you? What do you dislike (if anything) about it? Once you start answering these questions, you'll be well on your way to creating an amazingly satisfying sex life.

Probably right about now, though, you're thinking, "Who is Michael Thomas Ford and why is he talking to me about my sex life?" Good question. No, I'm not a doctor or a sex therapist or an educator with lots of initials after my name and diplomas from snooty schools hanging on my walls. I'm not even a porn star or sex worker. I'm just a regular guy. A guy more or less like you. I've *had* sex, so I do know a thing or two about it, and I've certainly talked about it a lot with other guys, so I know what we think about and worry about and want to understand when it comes to sex. Oh, yeah, and I've written about it quite a bit. If you've read any of the five essay collections in my *Trials of My Queer Life* series then you've read some of my thoughts about sex. And if you've read about some of my own disastrous sexual experiences that I write about in those titles you might be thinking it's a good idea to put this book down and look for another one. But I hope you won't, because there's some good stuff in here.

In addition to those publications I've also written some other things that are more advice-oriented. My book *100 Questions & Answers About AIDS: What You Need To Know Now*, for example, is one of the most widely used titles in HIV/AIDS education programs. Also, for a number of years I wrote (under different names) the popular "Sexpert" and "Sex Adviser" columns for *FreshMen* and *Men* magazines.

During that period of time I answered lots of questions about sex, relationships, aging, finding lovers, coming out, and the many assorted issues related to these things. And I wrote similar columns for other magazines as well.

So you see, I do have a little professional experience in this area. But for all the knowledge I possess in the field of sex, the most important factor is that I'm still a guy more or less like you. I've experienced a lot of the things we'll discuss in this book, and the things I haven't experienced I've researched and talked to other people about to find the answers. I want you to have a healthy sex life because that's a part of an overall

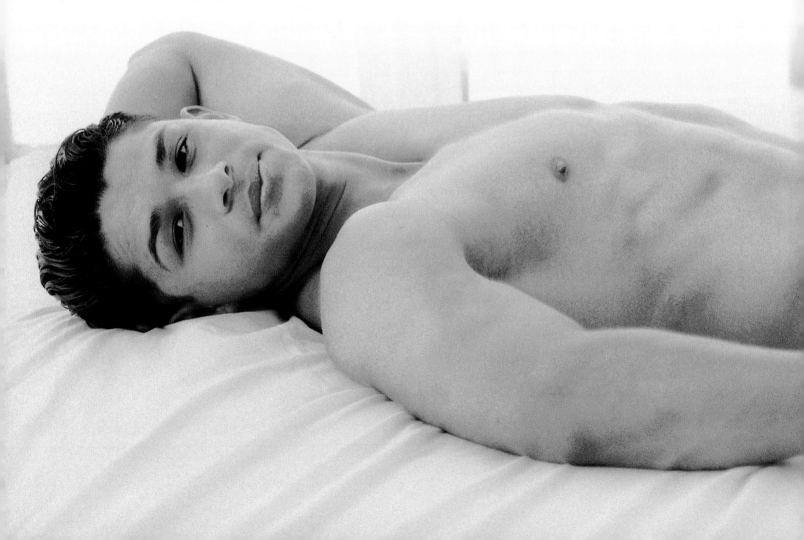

healthy and satisfying life. And I think you'll have a lot more fun discussing this kind of stuff with me than you would with someone else.

An interviewer once asked me why I include sex scenes as integral parts of my novels, the implication being that it's, well, sort of tacky. I answered, "Because writing is about capturing life, and sex is an important part of our lives." I really believe that. Our sex lives reflect other aspects of our lives, and in our sex lives we're free to explore who we are as men and who we are as sexual beings. If we don't talk about sex, we're ignoring a big part of who

we are as men and as people. And if we pretend that sex should be hidden away or relegated to "dirty" magazines and books, then we're only giving credence to all those old, damaging, and judgmental notions about sex that too many of us grew up with. So forget all about that. We're here to talk about sex. What do you want to know?

Michael Thomas Ford

Michael Thomas Ford

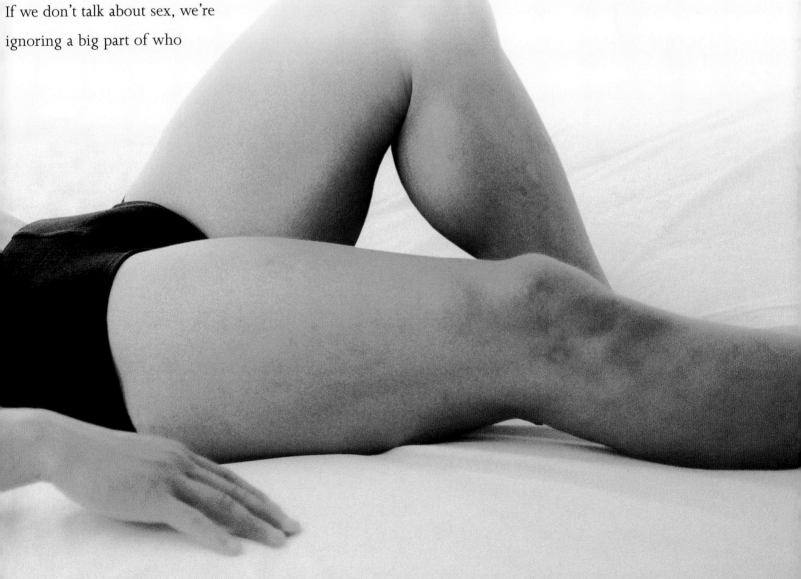

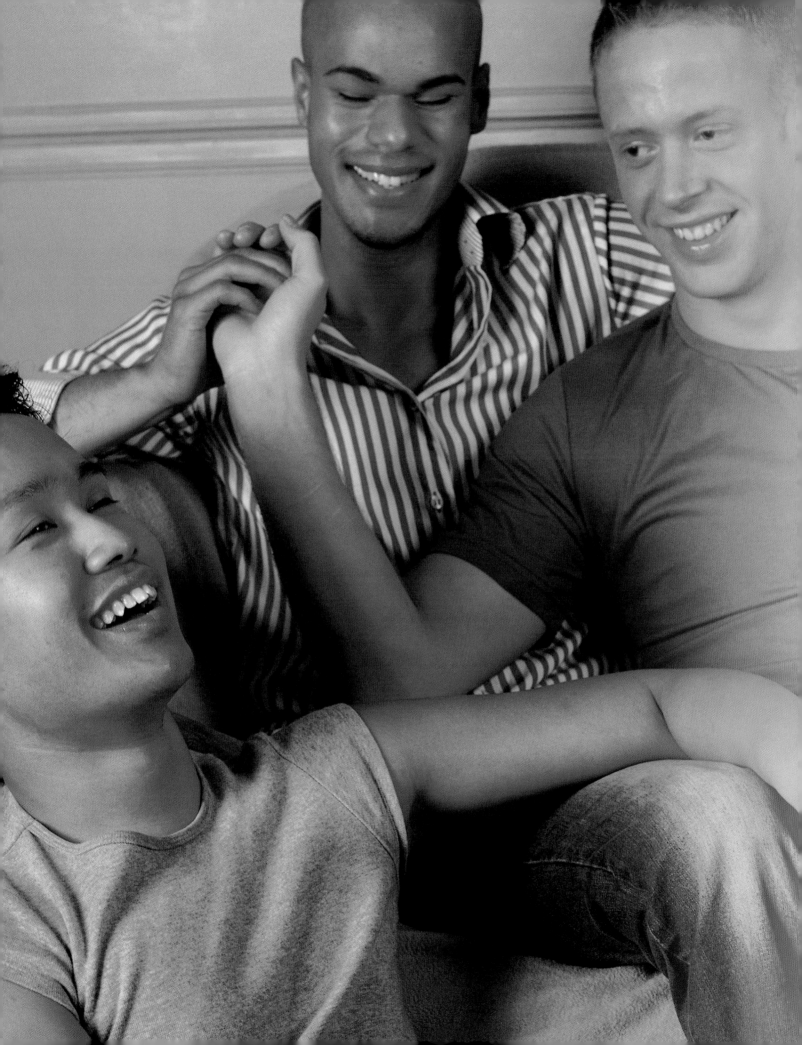

1 Being gay

What does it mean to be a gay man? What does it mean to be part of the gay world? The answers to these questions are different for each of us. How you see yourself as an individual, and as a member of a larger community, depends on many things, and there's no right or wrong way to be.

Straight men, gay men, and bisexuality

Examining why we are who we are

In 1948, pioneering sex researcher Alfred Kinsey published *Sexual Behaviour in the Human Male*, the results of the first comprehensive study of male sexuality. He then developed a numeric system of categorizing sexual behavior on a continuum, from exclusively heterosexual (1) to exclusively homosexual (6). Those whose sexual behaviors and attractions fell somewhere between 1 and 6 on the Kinsey Scale would be considered, to varying degrees, bisexual, or capable of being erotically aroused by either men or women. From his findings, Kinsey deduced that surprisingly few people were purely 1s or 6s, and that the range of human sexual behavior was far more complex than previously believed.

Each to his own

We can't always predict who we will find attractive and, what's more, our sexual and romantic inclinations may not be constant. How we identify ourselves and others sexually is not always as simple as it might seem. While many men identify themselves as either exclusively straight or exclusively gay, there are men whose sexuality is less well-defined. Some of these are men—partnered or single—who primarily have relationships with women, but also occasionally enjoy sex with other men. Others are men who

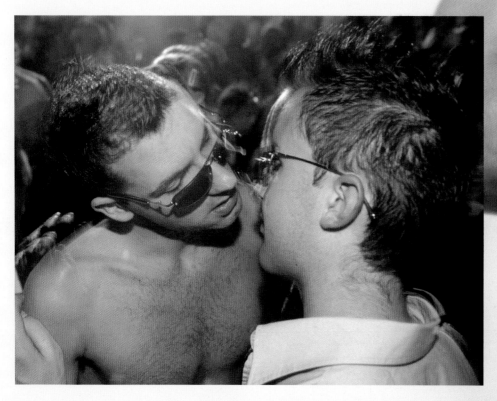

WHO YOU FIND yourself attracted to can sometimes surprise you, but allowing yourself to explore your feelings can result in unexpectedly fulfilling relationships.

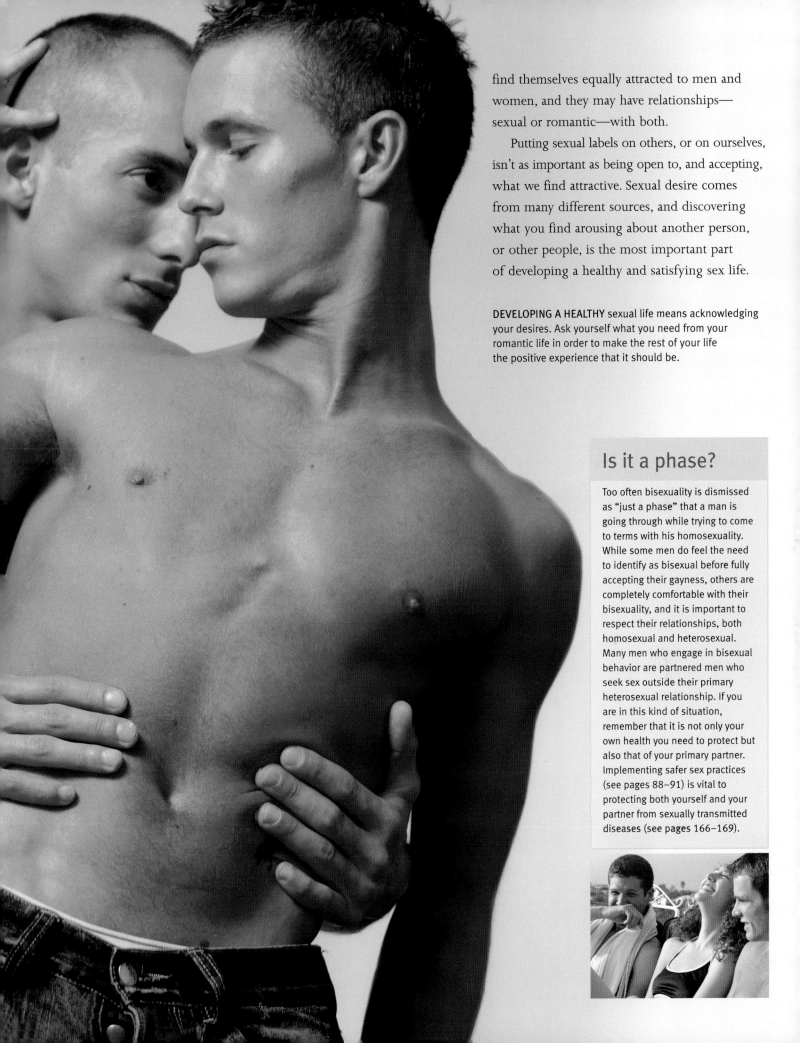

find themselves equally attracted to men and women, and they may have relationships—sexual or romantic—with both.

Putting sexual labels on others, or on ourselves, isn't as important as being open to, and accepting, what we find attractive. Sexual desire comes from many different sources, and discovering what you find arousing about another person, or other people, is the most important part of developing a healthy and satisfying sex life.

DEVELOPING A HEALTHY sexual life means acknowledging your desires. Ask yourself what you need from your romantic life in order to make the rest of your life the positive experience that it should be.

Is it a phase?

Too often bisexuality is dismissed as "just a phase" that a man is going through while trying to come to terms with his homosexuality. While some men do feel the need to identify as bisexual before fully accepting their gayness, others are completely comfortable with their bisexuality, and it is important to respect their relationships, both homosexual and heterosexual. Many men who engage in bisexual behavior are partnered men who seek sex outside their primary heterosexual relationship. If you are in this kind of situation, remember that it is not only your own health you need to protect but also that of your primary partner. Implementing safer sex practices (see pages 88–91) is vital to protecting both yourself and your partner from sexually transmitted diseases (see pages 166–169).

Coming out

Having the conviction to be you

What does coming out have to do with sex? A lot. The process of coming out helps you become a whole person. Hiding your sexuality requires a great deal of emotional effort, and the result can be that you don't feel free to express and explore who you are. With that pressure removed, you're able to live life openly and can more easily focus on creating a well-rounded life that includes healthy sex and relationships. The same is true for your partners. Dating or being in a relationship with someone who isn't out can create problems that affect the quality of these relationships.

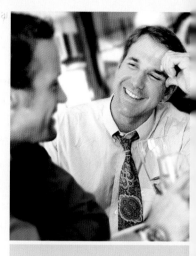

Circle of friends

If you're considering coming out, the most important thing you can do is establish a support network. This may consist of close friends or family you know you can count on. It can also be a more organized coming-out support group, perhaps at a gay community center. Or you may want to seek the help of a therapist or counselor who specializes in working with gay men who are coming out. There are numerous choices, so go for it!

Something you need to say

When we think about coming out, we envision breaking the news to our families and close friends. But that's only part of what coming out is. In a larger sense it's about accepting who we are as gay men and allowing ourselves to live our lives openly and fully. When we do that, other aspects of coming out (such as actually telling

our families and friends) are made easier and actually seem far less important than they do when we focus on them exclusively.

Most of us go through a period when, for various reasons, we're not out. Perhaps we're married, we're unsure of our sexuality, or we're living in a situation where coming out could be dangerous. Whatever the reason, keeping our sexuality hidden is, or seems to be, vitally important. During this time, exploring our

THE FIRST STEP in coming out is telling a close friend or a trusted member of your family. Be sure to give people time to absorb the news, and their support won't be far behind.

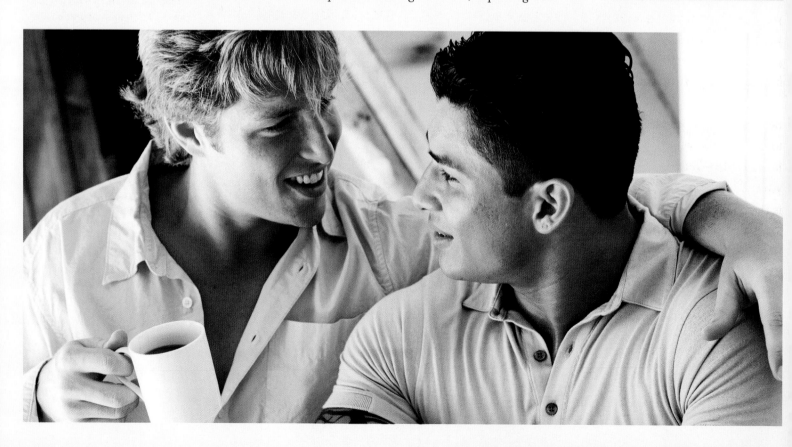

sexuality is limited by what kinds of risks we're willing to take. Perhaps we limit our sexual behavior to anonymous encounters or one-night stands (always at the other guy's place). Maybe we engage in sex only when we're traveling, to avoid running into anyone we know. Possibly we do actually become involved in a relationship, but we don't tell our families or anyone who might reveal our secret.

These are not healthy situations to find ourselves in. When any level of fear is involved in an activity, we aren't able to enjoy it fully. If we're constantly afraid that someone will "find out" about us, we can't really explore sexual or romantic relationships in the ways that we need to for them to enrich our lives. There's always going to be some measure of holding back, of keeping a part of ourselves out of the situation in case we have to make a hasty retreat.

A clear conscience

By coming out, you remove a great many of the obstacles to achieving sexual and romantic happiness. If you don't have anything to hide, you don't have anything to worry about. When you're free to explore what you like and who you like to do it with, you're free to develop into the man you want to be.

This isn't to say that coming out is necessarily right for everyone, or that you need to do it immediately. You might very well be in a situation that requires you to be discreet in your sexual behavior. Deciding when the time is right to come out is an individual matter. Some guys do it as soon as they are living on their own and are not dependent on anyone else. Others do it in steps, coming out to a few people at first and gradually increasing the circle of people with whom they interact as gay men.

The important thing is that you acknowledge who you are first, that you accept yourself and commit yourself to developing as a gay person and as a man. When you commit to that process, the other things fall into place. Sure, some of

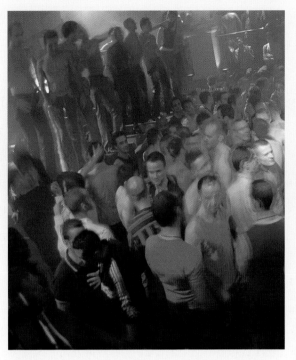

SOCIALIZING WITH other gay people reminds you that you are not alone in the world, and creates feelings of acceptance and support that strengthen your self-esteem.

them are harder than others. But if you're truly determined to live your life to the fullest, you'll know when the time is right.

Helping others to come out

Along the way you may find yourself dealing with a partner who isn't out yet. This can be difficult, particularly if it requires you to lie about your relationship or hide it at inconvenient times (such as when his parents or friends visit). In these situations you have to make a choice. Is being with this person helping you achieve what you want from your life, or is it holding you back? Are you comfortable rearranging your life to accommodate the needs of your partner?

You may find that you can accept the limitations of being with someone who isn't out, but you may also feel that it isn't working for you. Again, the important thing is that you focus on your life and make it what you want it to be. This may mean making some hard decisions about who you're with, but ultimately your happiness will depend on whether you do what's right for you, and not for someone else.

Step by step

Coming out is not a simple, single act, but rather a set of actions that results in living life openly as a gay man. Your own coming out process may consist of one or more of the following:

• **COMING OUT OF YOURSELF** Deciding that you're ready to live your life as a gay man is the most important step in coming out. It means you've accepted who you are and understand that it's an important aspect of becoming who you want to be.

• **COMING OUT TO FRIENDS** Most of us first come out to a close friend we know (or hope) will be supportive. If your friends react negatively, then keep in mind that it's because of *their* fears and misconceptions, and this response has nothing to do with you.

• **COMING OUT TO FAMILY** This is the one outing that causes the most anxiety for many of us. In reality, it's usually a lot easier than you think it's going to be. Even if your family reacts badly at first, giving them a little time usually helps them remember that you're the same person they've always known and loved.

• **COMING OUT TO THE WORLD** It sounds like a bigger deal than it really is. What this means is incorporating the rest of your life into the coming-out process, maybe by coming out at work or, say, with your soccer team, by joining a gay-related group, or becoming more involved in your local community.

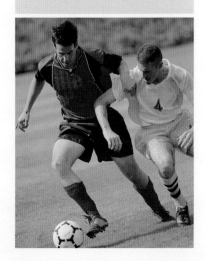

Gay image
Perceptions and misconceptions

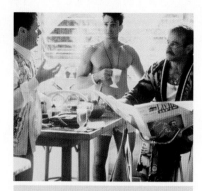

If you ask a dozen people to describe what a gay man looks or acts like, you'll get a dozen different answers. One may describe a good-looking guy with refined taste and perfect style, while another envisions a flamboyant character with outrageous mannerisms and a penchant for show tunes and gossip. Still others might tell you that gay men look and act "just like everyone else." The point is that every description is going to be correct because gay men come in all shapes, sizes, types, and styles. Despite media and cultural stereotypes, we aren't packaged in just one or two varieties.

In the beginning

When I was growing up the role models we had as gay men were largely limited to the Village People and, well, the Village People. There were men who people *thought* might be gay—Elton John and Rock Hudson, for example—but none of them were out, so we didn't know for certain. Even the Village People played it straight, as much as they could, for oblivious heterosexual fans. It was all a little confusing.

This was the age of the clone, the flannel-wearing, hairy-chested, mustachioed macho man who defied the stereotype of the gay man as a sissy. Many of us thought this was our only option as gay men, and if it didn't fit who we were or what we looked like, then we were out of luck. Fortunately for everyone, things have changed dramatically in the quarter century since the Village People taught us how to dress and flaunt ourselves (while singing along to *YMCA,* of course).

Now "being" gay isn't a matter of trying to look or act any one way. Sure, there are the gym bunnies who affect a particular physique, and perhaps a way of dressing, but that's always been

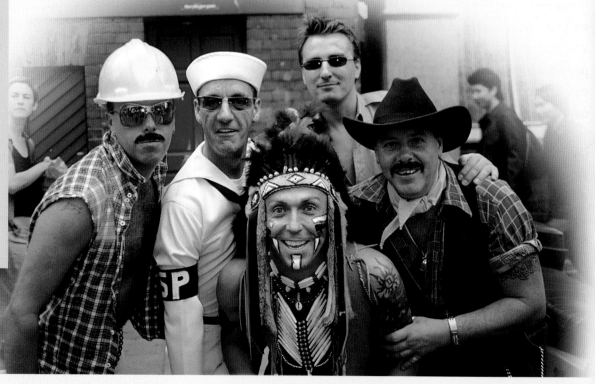

GAY IMAGE INCLUDES a wide range of styles, from the campy (such as the "Village People," shown here) to the serious, reflecting the diversity of the gay community.

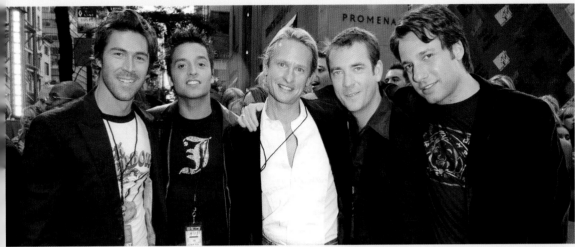

TELEVISION SHOWS such as *Queer Eye for the Straight Guy* have helped introduce gay culture—and gay people—to mainstream audiences.

Just as important as how gay people are portrayed in film is how we're portrayed in the media. Gay issues—particularly the issue of gay marriage—have become increasingly central to discussions of society and politics, and the way in which gay people are viewed is in large part a result of how our lives, our concerns, and our community as a whole are presented. For example, where media coverage of Gay Pride events or gay political actions once focused almost exclusively on the most dramatic aspects of gay culture, coverage now includes a more well-rounded view of who we are, which allows people to see past any misconceptions.

true, and not just in gay culture. For the most part, though, gay men are free to act and look however they please.

Now that we've evolved a little more in our thinking, we frequently go out of our way to tell people, particularly young gay men, that no, gay men aren't effeminate or bad at sports or fond of opera and ballet. And often that's true. But sometimes it is true, and trying to bury that truth is just as potentially damaging as the notion that all gay men are that way.

As a gay man, you have the right to explore who you are, wherever it might take you. Worrying about whether your interests and passions fit into someone else's idea of what you "should" be like only limits your own development as a man and as a person.

Sometimes being gay can feel like being in high school. Do I have the right clothes? Is this haircut okay? Why is his body better than mine? We compare ourselves to other men, and if we feel we're not as accomplished, stylish, or successful, we can get down on ourselves.

Deep down, very few of us ever really feel that we've gotten it all right. But I have news. You don't have to get it right. Today being gay means nothing and it means everything. It means you share one fundamentally important thing with a lot of other people. But sharing that

one thing also frees you up to become whoever and whatever you want to. More and more we discover gay people popping up in every single area of life. We're in the arts, politics, business, sports, medicine. We're in blue-collar jobs and white-collar careers. We truly are everywhere. Of course, some of the stereotypes are still popular. As our lives are portrayed more often on television and in film, we see that the image of the funny, sophisticated gay man still exists. That's okay. It's a positive image, and as gay people and gay lives become more and more a part of the larger culture, we'll see ourselves portrayed in a wider variety of ways that reflect the diversity that exists in our community.

Ultimately what's important is not what other people think we're like but what we really *are* like. And the more we express ourselves as individuals, the more difficult it will become for anyone—gay or straight—to try to force us into any definition or category.

THE IMAGE YOU project should be based on who you are, not on anyone else's idea of what you should be.

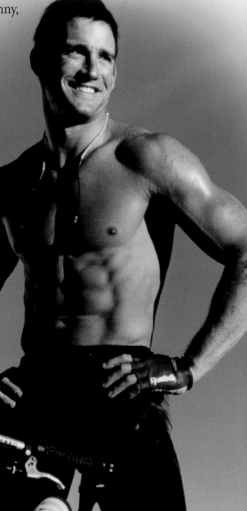

Diversity

Embracing cultural differences

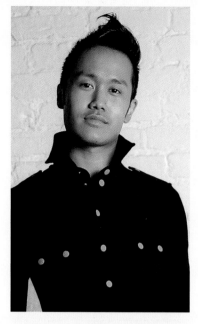

We all have various identities, whether we like them or not. Some of these we can change, some of these we can't. Identities are based on where we come from, what our professions are, where we went to school, what sports and hobbies we participate in, and many other things besides. We're Irish, and Russian, and Japanese. We're librarians, truck drivers, and landscapers. No matter who we are or where we come from, our differences both define us as unique and, at the same time, give us opportunities to be part of a wide range of groups, each of which shares certain bonds.

A shared experience

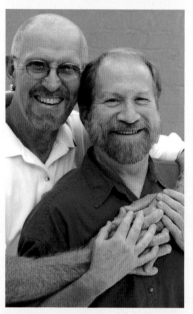

Being gay is unique because it encompasses *all* of these things. We can be gay *and* Italian, gay *and* soccer fans, gay *and* guys who ride Harleys. But no matter who we are, we're connected to everyone else who shares the trait of being gay.

This all makes for an incredibly diverse community of people; a massive, richly textured patchwork of guys who are sometimes at odds with one another. But even when we disagree, we still have that one thing that makes us family. Drag queens, gym rats, circuit queens, everyday Joes—we may be completely different from each other, but we have a shared experience, the experience of living in the world as gay men.

As gay people become more and more a visible part of society as a whole, the definition of "being gay" changes, and for the better. Although being gay is a common bond that unites us, we aren't all one type, as perceptions might have once suggested. We don't all look or act the same way. We're individuals, each with a unique life and a different story to tell. People can't just stick us in a category called "gay" and have that define us.

And neither should we. Be proud of being gay, and being part of the gay community, but be equally proud of everything else you are. The more you explore *all* of your identities, the more rewarding your life will be.

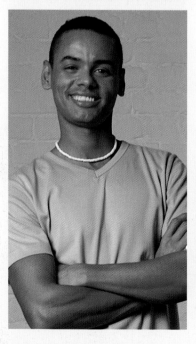

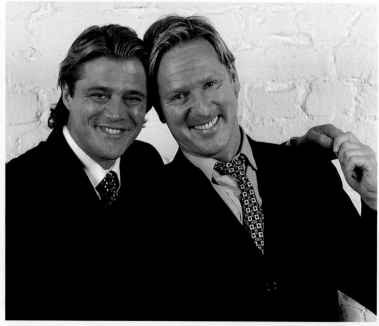

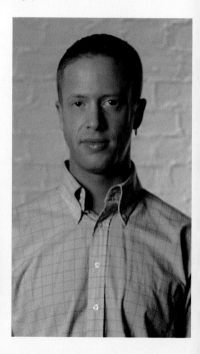

We are family

It's nice to think that because we're all gay we're all one big happy family. But really, like all families, we can sometimes be the littlest bit dysfunctional. We don't always find the same things important or want to help each other out with our causes. We bicker and fight over issues we disagree on. That's what all families do. But we also need to remember that we live in this world together, and that sometimes we need to help each other out, even if we don't particularly want to. Try to listen to other people and understand where they're coming from and why they're concerned with certain issues. What goes around comes around—and some day you might want them to help *you*.

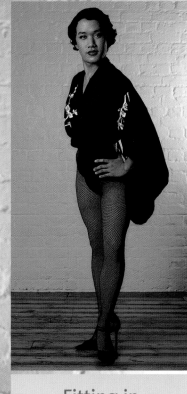

Fitting in

Finding your place in the gay community isn't always easy. The trick is to explore groups that interest you. There are groups for pretty much everything: athletes, leathermen, drag queens, seniors, teens, dads, pagans, just to name a few. Look for one that appeals to you and attend a meeting. It might take a couple of tries, but eventually you'll feel right at home.

THERE IS NO one way for gay men to look. The beauty of the gay community comes from the diverse faces of the people who are a part of it.

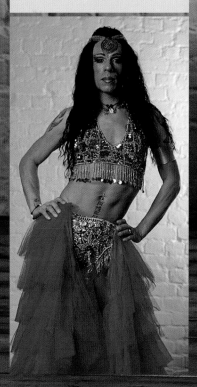

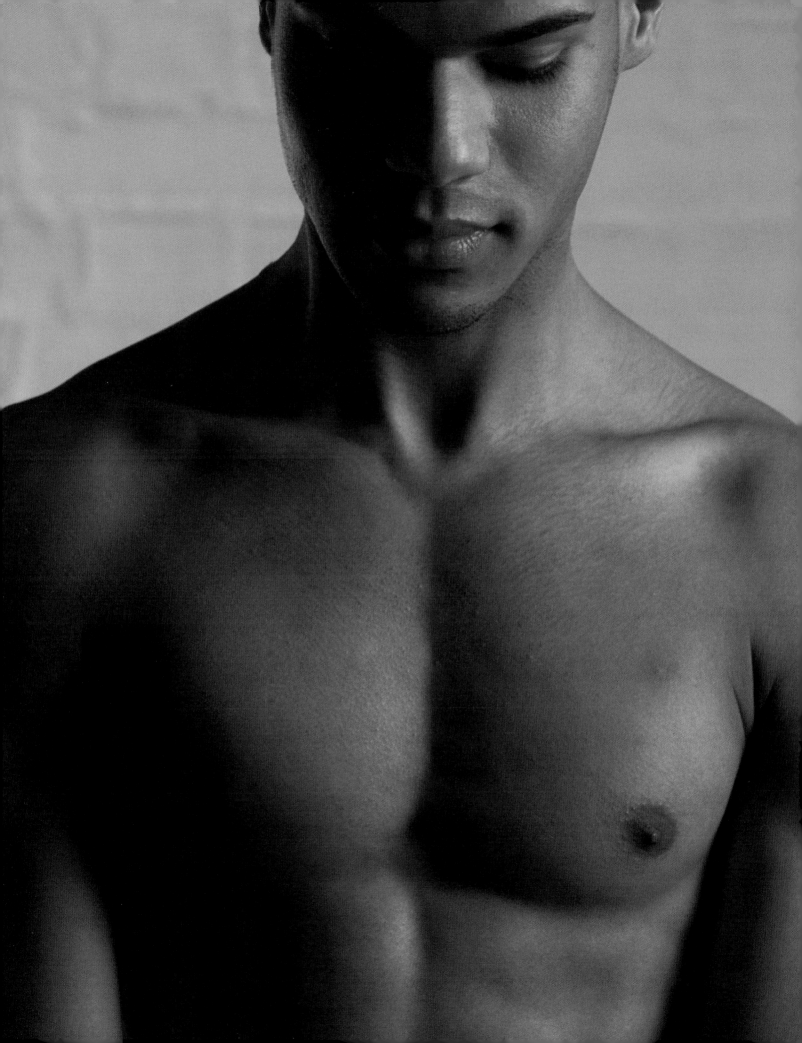

2 Your amazing body

The human body contains a universe of possibilities
for sexual enjoyment, and exploring the ways in
which you can give and receive pleasure is a
lifelong adventure. Knowing where to start, and
understanding how your body works, are the keys
to unlocking your sexual potential, and to creating
a sex life that grows with you and becomes richer
with each new experience.

Anatomy

Our bodies and what they do

Most of us are pretty aware of where the major parts of our bodies are. But not all of us are as knowledgeable about how these parts work and what roles they play when it comes to sex. So before we get into any details about what we can do with our bodies (or with a partner's body) we're going to have a little anatomy review, with particular emphasis on the parts we use the most when we get sexual. You might find some of this information easier to absorb if you take a look at your own equipment and follow along.

A little biology

Men come in all shapes and sizes, but when it comes to the inner workings of our bodies we're all pretty much alike. This is good news because it means that if you understand how your own body works, you understand how your partners' bodies work. Although there are individual variations, a penis is a penis, an anus is an anus, and they all work more or less the same. Spending some time learning how these things operate, and how you use them to create pleasure, will put you at the head of the class when it comes to sex.

Because the penis and the rectum are the principal players in most sexual activity, we're going to concentrate on them. Let's start with the penis. Take a look at the diagram. The penis is basically a sponge-filled tube. Not particularly sexy, is it? Well, at least it helps you understand what happens when you get hard. When you become aroused all of that spongy tissue fills up with blood, which is what causes the penis to stiffen and stand out from the body. When the blood has trouble reaching the tissue or staying in it, that's when we encounter erection difficulties (see pages 162–163).

What makes physical contact with the penis so arousing is the nerves that crowd this sensitive area, particularly the head of the penis. Having these nerve endings stimulated heightens sexual excitement and brings about ejaculation.

In ejaculation, sperm produced by the testicles and stored in the epididymis travel through the vas deferens to the seminal vesicle. Muscular contractions release the sperm and seminal fluid (produced by the prostate gland) into

(see pages 162–163)

Big deal?

Without a doubt, the number one concern men have about sex is the size of their penis. We worry about whether ours is too small, too big, too thick, not thick enough, oddly shaped, and all kinds of other things. So what's the truth?

The truth is that we each have our own idea of the perfect penis, and it's usually based on what we like, not on what we have ourselves. Studies show that the average erect penis is 5.2 inches long. But does it matter? No. A penis of any size or shape can get the job done.

You can't concern yourself with the size of your penis, otherwise it will affect your performance. What you *can* do is learn how to be a great lover. Then it won't matter to your partners what size you are.

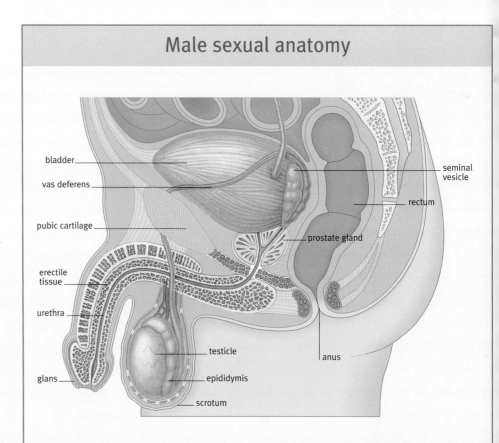

Male sexual anatomy

bladder
vas deferens
pubic cartilage
erectile tissue
urethra
glans
scrotum
testicle
epididymis
seminal vesicle
rectum
prostate gland
anus

The majority of the male sex organs are internal. The spongy tissue of the penis produces erections when filled with blood, and the testicles, epididymis, vas deferens, prostate gland, seminal vesicles, and urethra are all involved in the process of ejaculation.

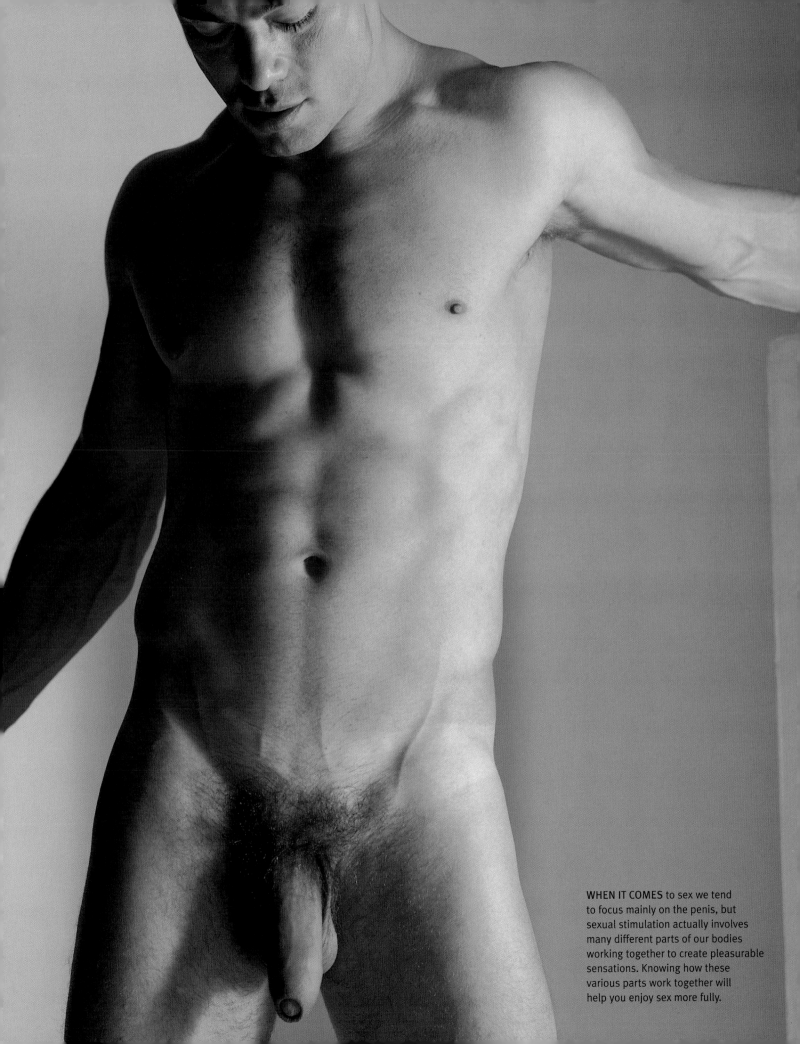

WHEN IT COMES to sex we tend to focus mainly on the penis, but sexual stimulation actually involves many different parts of our bodies working together to create pleasurable sensations. Knowing how these various parts work together will help you enjoy sex more fully.

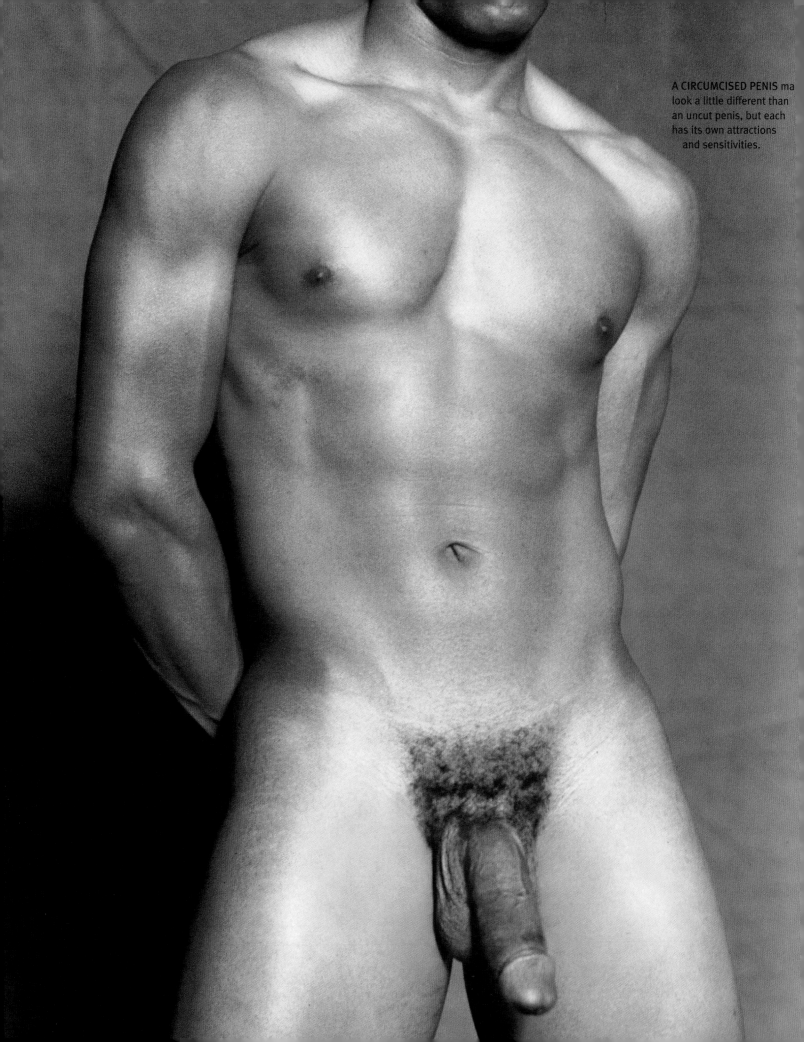

A CIRCUMCISED PENIS ma
look a little different than
an uncut penis, but each
has its own attractions
and sensitivities.

Cut vs uncut

No matter where you go or what you may have heard, penises are mostly alike. The only real difference you may encounter is between a circumcised (cut) and uncircumcised (uncut) partner.

Circumcision is an operation in which the foreskin is removed from the penis. Some cultures believe that the foreskin is redundant and gets in the way of good hygiene. Others are of the opinion that it is a very sensitive and vital part of the male anatomy that shouldn't be removed.

Men who are uncut sometimes require extra care. The foreskin should slide easily over the head, but sometimes it can be rather tight. Pulling on or forcing your partner's foreskin away from the head will create discomfort, so be careful.

In addition, men who are uncut are sometimes more sensitive to stimulation of the penis head. Again, to avoid causing any pain, be very careful when sucking, stroking, or otherwise stimulating an uncut partner.

Although foreskins may require additional cleaning, it isn't true that uncut penises are naturally dirty or smelly, so don't let that misconception influence your attitude toward uncircumcised men. We're all the same in the end!

the urethra, where they mix and create semen (cum). The semen is then pumped through the urethra and out of the penis.

Probing deeper

Not too difficult to understand, right? Well, the rectum is even easier. If you look at the diagram of the male sexual anatomy on page 22, you'll see that the anus is the entrance to the rectum (which is actually the end of the large intestine). The opening and closing of the anus is controlled by the sphincter muscle, which is a band of muscle that surrounds the anus. The rectum itself is comprised of a thin membrane.

During sexual activity involving the rectum, objects (fingers, a penis, a dildo, or other sex toy) are generally pushed through the anus and into the rectum. Any pain that accompanies this kind of activity is almost always a result of pushing against the sphincter muscle, which normally remains tightly closed. This is why it's so important to relax that muscle and to use lubricant to ensure smooth entry.

Understanding how the sphincter works is particularly important to enjoying anal sex. If you spend some time getting to know your own, you'll get a feel (literally) for what it does. Use your fingers to experience how the sphincter expands and contracts, and note what makes you tense up and what makes

you relax. When you learn how to control the sphincter muscle, and how to make your partners relax, you'll be well on your way to having enjoyable anal sex.

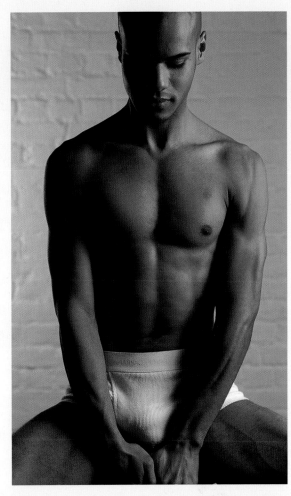

TAKE TIME TO explore your own body, and learn how you respond to various types of stimulation. This will make it easier to communicate your desires to your partners, plus you'll have a better idea of what they enjoy.

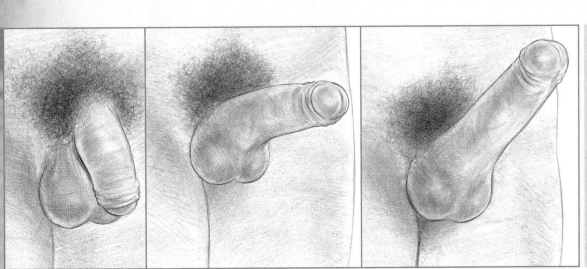

The erection

• Normally the penis hangs between the legs, testicles relaxed.

• During arousal, blood rushes into the tissue of the penis, causing it to stiffen. The glans (head of the penis) swells with blood.

• At full erection, the scrotum thickens, the head of the penis swells and darkens to a deep red or purplish color, and the testicles may draw up closer to the body.

Erogenous zones

The subjects of touch

Named after the Greek god of love, Eros, erogenous zones are areas of the body that, when physically stimulated, initiate or enhance sexual arousal. The most obvious are in particularly sensitive areas where there are concentrations of nerve endings, such as around the nipples and the genitals, but for many people the ears, feet, mouth, and buttocks, are also highly sensual. In fact, any part of the body can be an erogenous zone if stimulating it is sexually exciting, and discovering which areas turn your lover (and you) on is all part of the fun of lovemaking.

The pleasure principle

Too often when we think about making love we concentrate only on what happens with and to our genitals. In reality, the entire body has the potential to provide pleasure. Try rubbing the back of the neck, gently biting a nipple, running a finger along the spine. All of these actions can heighten sexual excitement.

By stimulating various parts of the body, you can initiate action or change the direction of action already taking place. You probably already know where some of your erogenous zones are

and what they feel like to touch. Do you go crazy when a lover runs his tongue down your neck? Does having your earlobe bitten send shivers down your spine? When a partner's fingers find their way between the cheeks of your ass, does a moan escape your lips? These are all common erogenous zones, and you've probably experienced having one or more of them aroused during sex.

But what about those erogenous zones that aren't so obvious? Does the idea of someone sucking your toes turn you on? How about

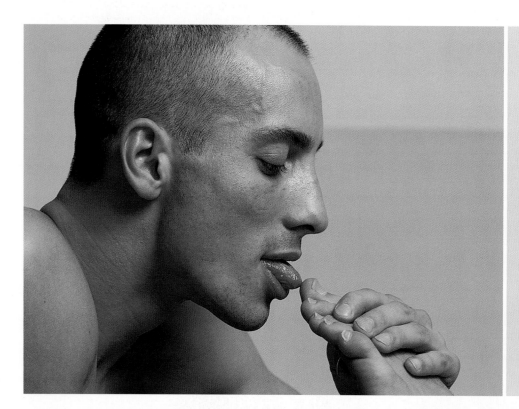

"Oh, yeah!" vs "Oh, no!"

There's a fine line between pleasure and pain. What makes you go "Mmm" may make your partner go "Ow!" Not everyone likes their nipples being pinched or played with, for example, and a tongue in the ear could make one guy squirm and another one go wild with ecstasy. The secret is to explore your partner's body with your eyes, hands, tongue, and anything else that feels good. Start slowly and see what kind of reactions you get when you pay attention to different areas of his body. Talk to him—you're not a mind reader! Ask him to tell you what he likes, and talk dirty to him—to make him even hornier.

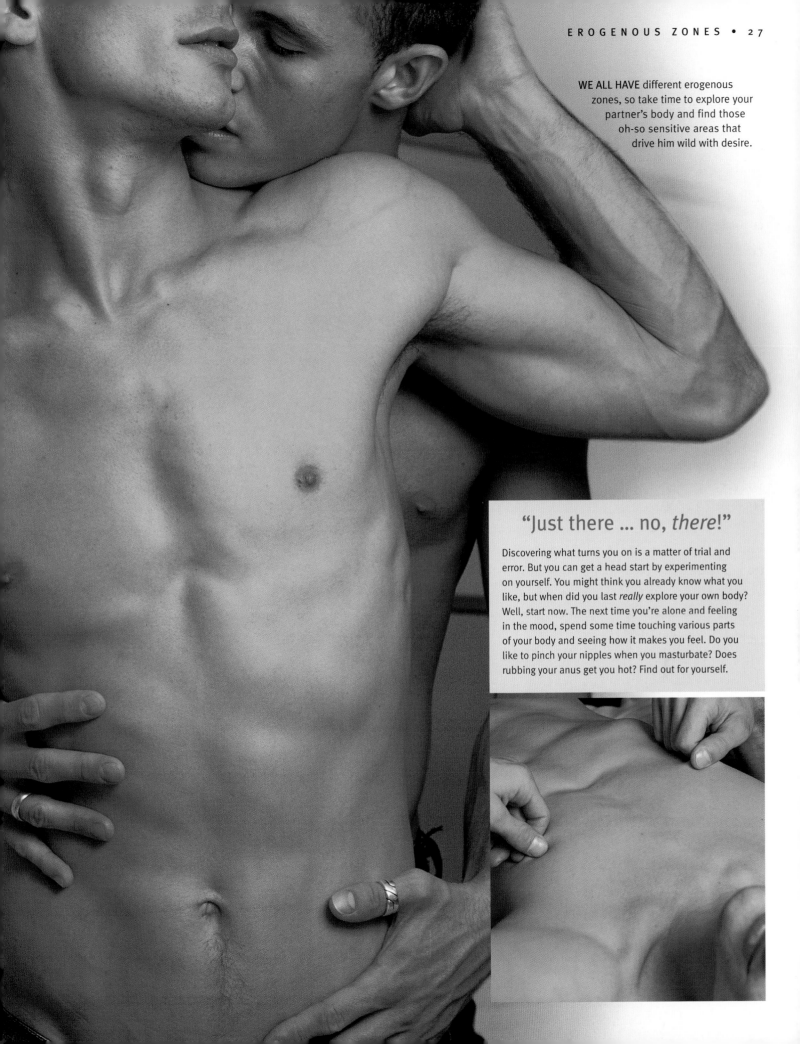

WE ALL HAVE different erogenous zones, so take time to explore your partner's body and find those oh-so sensitive areas that drive him wild with desire.

"Just there ... no, *there*!"

Discovering what turns you on is a matter of trial and error. But you can get a head start by experimenting on yourself. You might think you already know what you like, but when did you last *really* explore your own body? Well, start now. The next time you're alone and feeling in the mood, spend some time touching various parts of your body and seeing how it makes you feel. Do you like to pinch your nipples when you masturbate? Does rubbing your anus get you hot? Find out for yourself.

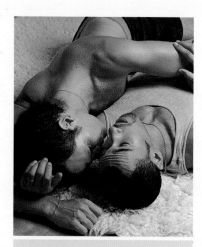

Clothes encounters

Naked or clothed? Sometimes it can be fun to see how much you can turn your partner on by focusing on the parts of his body you can touch when he has his clothes *on*. Stroking his hair and face, kissing the back of his neck, and playing with his fingers are all things you can do to stimulate sexual desire. Best of all, you can do these kinds of things in most public places, and they can be great ways to get each other worked up for the hot and sweaty action you've got planned for when you get home.

having your head rubbed or your navel tongued? Experiment with paying attention to different parts of the body and you just might be surprised to find where your pleasure spots are.

Ecstasy through exploration

The path you take on the journey around your partner's body depends on the circumstances. A kiss while you're sitting on the couch or standing in the kitchen gives you an opportunity to run your tongue over his neck, bite his ear, or run your hand up the back of his neck and into his hair. Any or all of these things may be just what it takes to get him going and the only way you'll find out is by trying. You can continue exploring his body as you help him remove his clothes. This undressing can be an incredibly sexy event all by itself, particularly if you take your time and stop every so often to enjoy the different stages of undress. Running your fingers over the bulge in his underwear before getting to what's underneath, for example, can be a real turn-on.

Once the clothes are off, you're really ready to go to town. Using your hands, mouth, and tongue, you can try stimulating your lover from head to toe. In fact, sometimes it's easiest literally

to start at the top and work your way down. Go from kissing to running your tongue over his chest and down into his crotch. Use your hands to stroke his penis and fondle his testicles. Dart your tongue into the sensitive area beneath the balls. Teasing his anus with your fingers or tongue can be particularly pleasurable.

The goal here is to heighten sexual excitement, so go slowly. Make your movements sensuous. Really focus on whatever body part or area you're working on and see what kinds of stimulation your partner likes. If he reacts to having his armpit licked, for example, give him more. If he responds to a tug on his testicles with a groan, be more aggressive in that area.

The same is true for you. If your partner is doing something that sends you gasping for air, let him know. A good loud moan should do the trick, and if he doesn't get the hint then gently pushing his head or hand back to the magic spot will do just fine.

THE NIPPLES ARE especially sensitive areas of the body. Some guys like a full-on nibble or even a bite, but others go crazy with just a flick of the tongue.

Erogenous moans—how to induce them

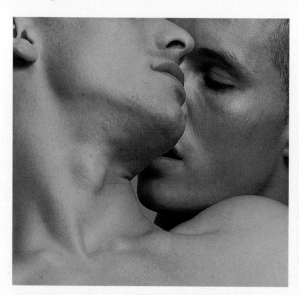

THE NECK and below the chin are particularly sensitive areas. Kissing or running your tongue over these parts is a great way to arouse or enhance sexual desire.

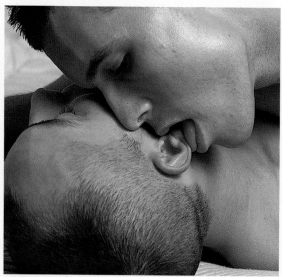

SOME MEN ENJOY having their ears nibbled or tongued. The trick is to do it gently and not slobber on your partner like a dog going at a bone.

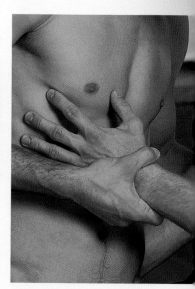

IF YOUR PARTNER guides your hands to a particular place on his body, take his hint and explore further.

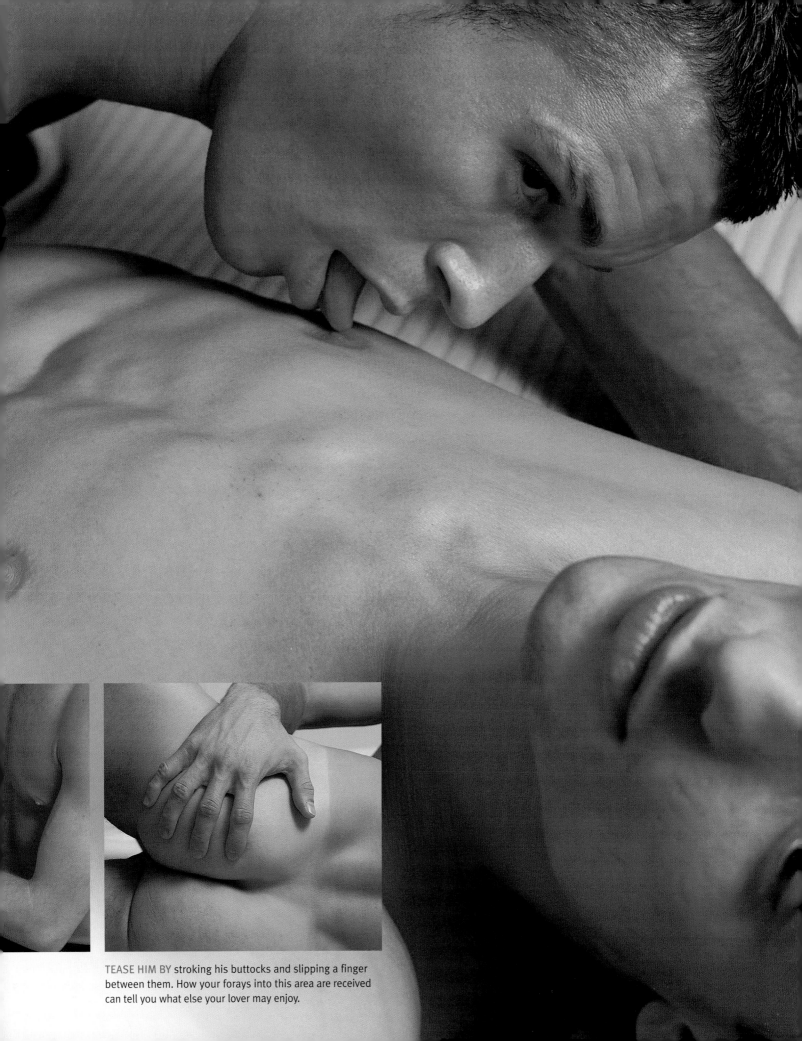

TEASE HIM BY stroking his buttocks and slipping a finger between them. How your forays into this area are received can tell you what else your lover may enjoy.

Sex and health

Looking after body and mind

A healthy sex life develops out of having an overall healthy lifestyle. When you feel well physically you also feel well mentally and emotionally, and when you feel confident about yourself you approach all aspects of your life with a more positive outlook. This doesn't mean that in order to have a satisfying sex life you have to be in perfect physical shape. It means maintaining a level of health and fitness that allows you to operate efficiently, inspires you to feel good about how you look, and encourages a positive mental state.

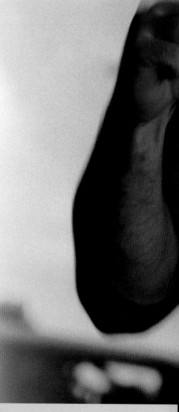

FIGHTING FIT Lack of physical exercise is detrimental to your health. Your libido, your waistline, and your cardiovascular fitness will all suffer unless you embark on a moderate exercise regime.

Just (health) checking

If you own a car then chances are you'll know how often you need to change the oil, check tire pressure, and have it serviced. But do you know how often you should have an all-over appraisal? We men tend to ignore warning signs about our health, only to discover serious illnesses when they have caused damage beyond repair. So start by making an appointment with your physician, have that check-up, and then make routine appointments to help keep your body and mind in top condition.

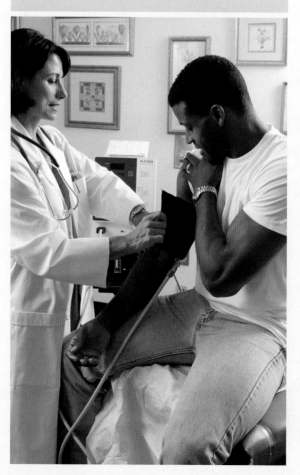

Great expectations

Gay culture is, unfortunately, sometimes far too obsessed with body image. The gay media is filled with images of men who have "perfect" bodies, much in the same way that the straight media is filled with images of women who are impossibly thin or who possess what are perceived as ideal dimensions. This simply confirms that the old adage "sex sells" is a true one.

But what else do these images sell? Sadly, the very images that are meant to attract and arouse us can also inflict deep emotional wounds. If we feel that we can never attain the look we're told is needed to be attractive to other men, it's easy to come to the false conclusion that we aren't worthy of having positive, satisfying sex lives. This negative attitude can quickly develop into other self-destructive behaviors. Just as many women develop eating disorders and other psychological issues as a result of feeling unattractive, eating disorders and depression centered around negative body image are becoming more and more common in gay men.

Dispelling a common myth

Here's a little secret: guys with great bodies don't always have great sex. It's true. The guys who have great sex are men who are simply happy with how they look and feel. Sure, they might want to lose 20 pounds, have more defined (or even remotely defined) abs, or get their ass back

Sex and steroids

In order to achieve the kind of sculpted bodies they want, some men resort to taking illegal steroids to enhance the effects of their workouts. Although steroids can indeed increase muscle mass, they can also have a negative effect on your sex life. In addition to causing changes in mood and behavior, they are also known to cause prostate enlargement, testicular atrophy, and sexual dysfunction.

Go to your happy place

Stress can be one of the biggest—and most overlooked—obstacles to achieving a satisfying sex life. Often we don't realize how much the pressures of daily life are wearing on us. Activities that focus on being more aware of the mind/body connection, such as meditation and yoga, can be wonderful tools for helping us let go of negative feelings and getting more in touch with our bodies.

to the way it looked when they were younger, but basically they're okay with their bodies. And because they're okay with how they look, this frees them up psychologically to concentrate on what really makes sex good, which is relating intimately to another person.

Being realistic

The fact is, most of us don't have the time it takes to develop the bodies portrayed in magazines or porn films. Frankly, there are many more useful ways to spend our time than going to the gym for several hours a day just to achieve a pumped-up chest or huge, rippling arms, and worrying about every piece of food we put in our mouths takes a great deal of the joy out of what should be a wonderful experience. Too many of us subject ourselves to emotional (and sometimes physical) torture just because we think we have to work toward a standard set by someone else.

This doesn't mean there's no need for going to the gym or taking that daily run if you want to. What it does mean is realizing that a healthy body is one that allows you to do the things you want to do, and to enjoy a well-rounded life.

Getting the balance right

So what *should* we be concerned about when it comes to sex and health? Regular exercise is important because it gives us energy and stamina, both of which play important roles in sex. But what that exercise consists of can vary greatly from man to man. For some of us a daily 15-minute walk is enough, while for others a 5-mile run or an hour on the treadmill are more appropriate. What you do depends on what you like, what your health goals are, and what you can comfortably do in the time you have. Again, look outside the gym. A weekly game of softball or soccer with your buddies is just as good, and probably more fun, than time spent lifting weights by yourself. Swimming, yoga, hiking, scuba diving, martial arts, skiing, and rock climbing will all get your body moving and provide additional benefits. Don't limit yourself by thinking that "working out" has to mean doing one thing.

What you put into your body also affects both how you look and feel. There are many different types of recommended dietary systems out there,

most of which completely contradict each other, so suggesting one eating plan for everyone is impossible. But in general it's important that you understand how what you eat affects you, both physically and emotionally. Sugar, for example, affects people differently, as do caffeine, red meat, carbohydrates, and many other things we consume on a regular basis. Eating certain things may make you feel depressed or tired, while others may help you feel energized and focused. So monitor the foods you eat and how they affect you.

Up in smoke

In addition to the foods we eat, other things we put into our bodies affect us emotionally and physically and have an impact on our sex lives. Although a few guys find smoking (particularly cigars) a turn-on, lighting up isn't going to help you out when it comes to getting it on. In addition to reduced lung capacity, arterial constriction, that attractive hacking, and a little thing called cancer, smoking has some

How can I stay in good shape?

Diets go in and out fashion, and magazines are full of conflicting advice on what we should or should not eat and drink. In fact, there is just one basic, simple principle to follow: Eat a varied and balanced diet of wholesome foods, including five portions of fruit and vegetables each day. Avoid convenience and processed foods as well as fatty or sweet snacks such as chocolate, cookies, and chips. Choose whole-grain, rather than white, bread, rice, and pasta. Eat plenty of oily fish such as sardines, salmon, and tuna, which are high in unsaturated fats.

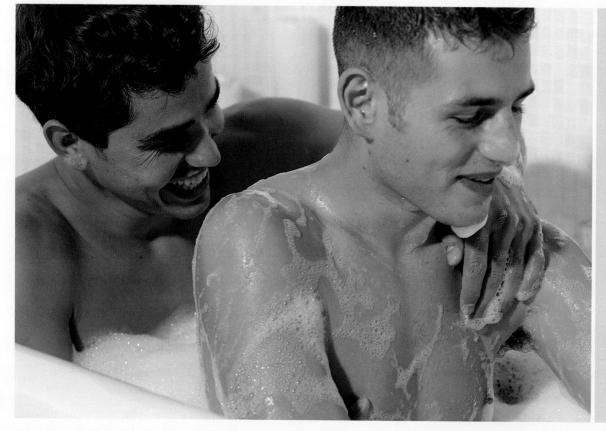

Hygiene tips

Being clean shouldn't be thought of as a lifestyle choice—it's a necessity. The following pointers will help you stay spotless:

• Bathe or shower once a day. You'll smell nice, and good personal hygiene can help cut down risks from bacterial infections.

• Be sure to keep your hair, nails, skin, and teeth clean. Healthy body, healthy mind.

• A daily shave is an easy way to make you look and feel refreshed. If you have facial hair, keep it neatly trimmed.

• Avoid overdoing it with colognes and other scents. Smells, even good ones, can be overpowering.

• Don't forget your teeth. Regular visits to the dentist will keep them looking great.

LET'S FACE IT, we all want to look good. Forget lifting weights—the first step to looking your best is diet. Watch those calories, choose a wide range of foods, and *enjoy* what you eat.

Sexercise

Did you know there's an exercise that can help you tighten the anus for an extra-sexy squeeze when your partner is inside? It's called the Pilates squeeze: First, lie face down on a comfortable surface and place a small pillow or cushion between your upper thighs. Rest your head on the back of your hands and put your toes together, keeping your heels apart. Then inhale and draw up your stomach muscles. Tighten your buttock muscles, squeeze the cushion between your inner thighs, and put your heels together. Count to five and release. Repeat this exercise ten times. After you've given yourself a little time to relax, start thinking about how great you'll feel the next time you have sex with your partner.

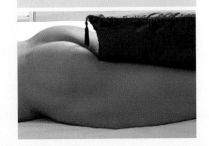

less deadly but still unpleasant effects. Skin discoloration, bad breath, and stained teeth are some of the more lovely reminders cigarettes leave behind. Oh, yeah, and if you need another reason to quit, smoking makes your dick and your cum taste awful.

There are more details about alcohol on pages 174–175, but it deserves mention here because alcohol abuse is one of the leading factors in sexual dysfunction. And don't forget the detrimental effect that drugs have on the body: Some people think that using stimulants such as Ecstasy and poppers increases sexual enjoyment, but in fact, these drugs can have a

potentially deadly, effect. Similarly, depressants such as alcohol can contribute to numerous physical health issues, as well as psychological problems, including loss of inhibition, which can contribute to participation in risky sexual activities.

Developing a healthy body and a healthy sex life really does depend on knowing exactly how your body is affected by what you put in it. Once you understand what that relationship is, you will develop a positive attitude toward diet and behavior that will reinforce all of your efforts, not only to be physically healthy, but to pursue relationships that are healthy as well.

Personal image

How you see yourself: How others see you

How you present yourself to the world has an enormous effect on how you're perceived by potential partners. Creating a positive personal image that reflects who you are as a man will help you make an engaging impression that attracts the kinds of men you want to attract. This image is a combination of physical appearance and mental attitude. The two need to work together in order to be successful, so learning how to make your outside appearance match your inner personality is the key to creating a winning overall image.

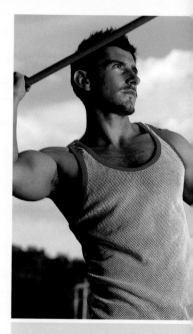

Be yourself

We all know really handsome men who never have successful relationships, and guys who don't have model good looks but who always seem to have dates. Sure, what you look like is important, but what's much more important is creating an overall package that appeals to the men you want to attract. Having a perfect body, handsome face, and stylish wardrobe may get you a lot of attention, but if there's nothing behind it, guys won't hang around for long.

Creating a personal image starts with figuring out who you are as a man. Too often gay men go for a look they see on other people, or that they think is what gay men are supposed to look like. If you want to bleach your hair, get a tribal tattoo, and walk around in a white tank top, that's fine. But before you go ahead and do so, make sure it's because it's really who you are and not because you're just imitating what everyone

else is doing. It's easy to look like everyone else, but being yourself—being unique—is ultimately going to be much more satisfying.

Gay men come in all kinds of packages. Trying to fit yourself into a package that isn't you is just going to make you uncomfortable. When creating your personal style, think about who you are. What do you like to do? What's special about you? What kind of image do you want to project?

Creating a look

Your clothes are a reflection of your tastes and interests, so use them to create a first impression. If you're a T-shirt-and-jeans kind of guy, go with that look. If you're more comfortable in trendy clothes, make that look work for you. The key is to be what you are and not what you aren't. Don't do the cowboy hat, boots, and

Body beautiful

Too many gay men suffer from a negative body image. Convinced by the media that we have to have perfect bodies in order to be attractive to other men, many of us subject ourselves to punishing workout routines, unhealthy diets, and even surgery and other extreme measures, in the hopes of achieving what we think is going to be the ideal body.

The truth is that a beautiful body is one that is healthy and allows us to do what we want to do. A beautifully muscled body can be a big component of physical attraction, but it's not the whole picture. Much more sexy is a body that performs well and reflects a man's overall lifestyle.

Rather than focus on developing perfect abs or a huge chest, work on making your body a healthy one. If this means getting yourself into the gym, fine, but don't let how you look become an obsession. Other men may be attracted to your body initially, but eventually they may figure out that it was only your face and physique that they had the hots for and not your mind.

CREATING YOUR OWN style begins with working out who you are. Once you feel confident about that, you will know what kind of overall image you want to project.

eans thing unless that's really the kind of guy you are. Don't cram yourself into clothes that aren't right for you simply because they look good on someone else. If you aren't comfortable in what you're wearing, it's going to show.

There's a truly unfortunate tendency in a lot of gay men to want to buy an image. This is best illustrated by the popularity of clothing designers and stores that sell particular looks. Rather than trying to create their own personal image, men attempt to purchase one by wearing certain labels. A store-bought image isn't going to fool anyone. Just because a shirt has a recognizable name on it, or a hat has someone's initial embroidered across it, doesn't make you special. In fact, wearing such clothing really just makes you look a little desperate and unoriginal. Avoid falling for false images. You don't want labels applied to you as a man, so why have them on your clothes?

THERE'S NO NEED to be obsessive about personal hygiene, but keeping yourself well-groomed is all part of making sure you are an attractive and pleasant guy to be with.

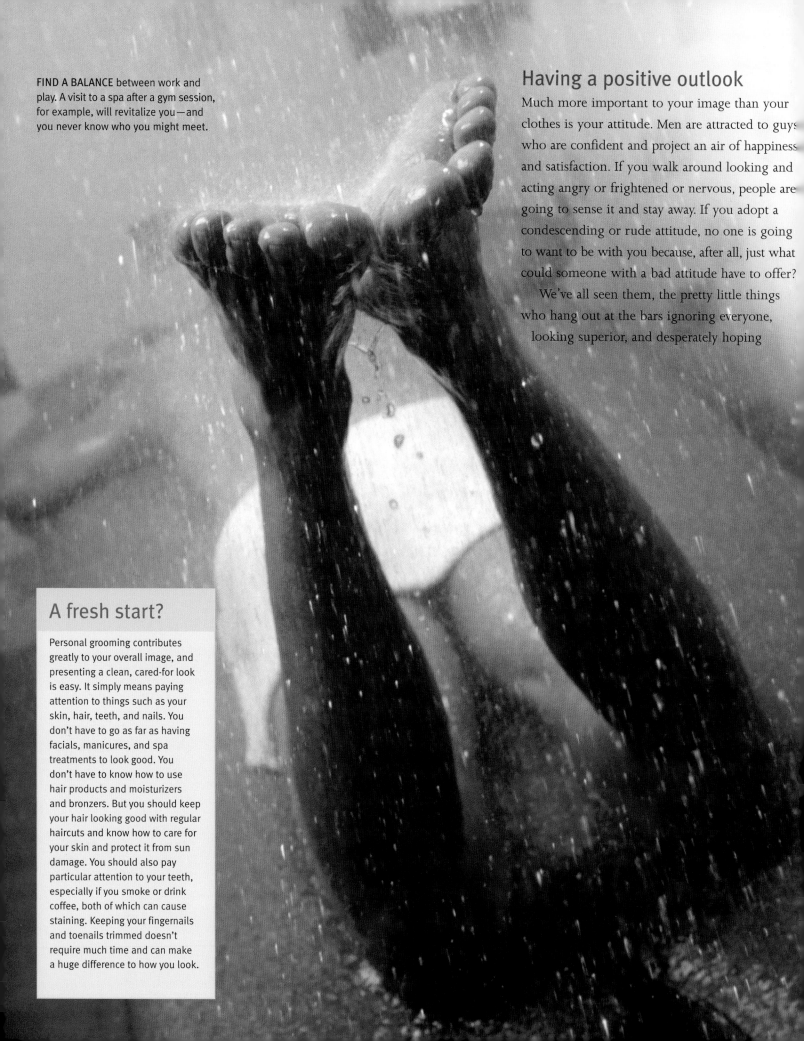

FIND A BALANCE between work and play. A visit to a spa after a gym session, for example, will revitalize you—and you never know who you might meet.

Having a positive outlook

Much more important to your image than your clothes is your attitude. Men are attracted to guys who are confident and project an air of happiness and satisfaction. If you walk around looking and acting angry or frightened or nervous, people are going to sense it and stay away. If you adopt a condescending or rude attitude, no one is going to want to be with you because, after all, just what could someone with a bad attitude have to offer?

We've all seen them, the pretty little things who hang out at the bars ignoring everyone, looking superior, and desperately hoping

A fresh start?

Personal grooming contributes greatly to your overall image, and presenting a clean, cared-for look is easy. It simply means paying attention to things such as your skin, hair, teeth, and nails. You don't have to go as far as having facials, manicures, and spa treatments to look good. You don't have to know how to use hair products and moisturizers and bronzers. But you should keep your hair looking good with regular haircuts and know how to care for your skin and protect it from sun damage. You should also pay particular attention to your teeth, especially if you smoke or drink coffee, both of which can cause staining. Keeping your fingernails and toenails trimmed doesn't require much time and can make a huge difference to how you look.

someone will come over and adore them. Sure, there are guys who find this kind of attitude intriguing, at least initially. But mostly these guys are going to attract other men with bad attitudes—which is probably a good thing, because they deserve each other.

But the men who will have real success are the ones who have open, friendly personalities. They're the guys who don't act superior to everyone around them, who don't treat people badly, and who don't whine and complain about things. There is nothing attractive about someone who is unhappy. You attract the same kind of energy that you put out, and a positive, outgoing guy is always going to be more attractive than someone who projects negativity.

Building a lifestyle

Your personal image extends into the whole of your life. It's comprised not just of what you look like but also of the activities you participate in and what you do with your time. If you spend all your nights in bars hoping someone great will come along, you're going to find yourself disappointed. But if you get out and participate in things you enjoy, you're going to make yourself happier and as a result be more attractive to others. So spend some time playing sports, volunteering, or just enjoying time with friends doing things you like. By doing these things you'll make yourself a happier person, and this will enhance the image you present to other people.

Making yourself a well-rounded man will also add to your personal image. The books you read, the music you listen to, the hobbies you enjoy, and the things you are able to talk about and express opinions on all make an impression on people. If the only topic of conversation you have is the weather, you're not going to make a very interesting dinner companion, are you? Ideas are sexy, and being able to converse on a variety of topics will make you a man people like spending time with.

Your home, too, is a reflection of you. Spend a bit of time making your house or apartment a welcoming place, a place where visitors will enjoy spending time with you. If you put a bit of attention and care into your personal surroundings, it will show. Create a space that actually says something about the man who lives in it, instead of being no more than a place where you store your belongings.

The complete package

All of these things—appearance, attitude, and lifestyle—are part of your personal image. The more complete you make this package, the more likely you are going to be to attract partners who are equally appealing. The more you succeed in projecting an accurate and interesting portrait of who you are as a man, the happier you're going to be, and this self-confidence is going to extend into your sexual and romantic relationships, too.

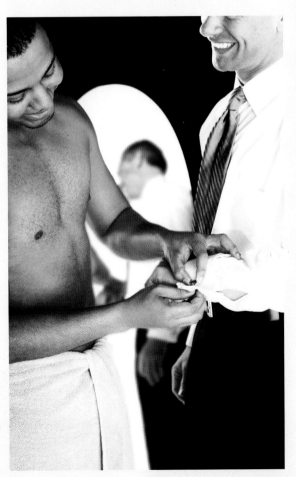

EXPRESS YOUR APPRECIATION of the way your partner takes care of his appearance by choosing his tie and helping him with the finishing touches of his outfit.

Home improvement

Making your home a reflection of yourself doesn't have to be difficult. Here are suggestions for a few simple things that you can do to create lasting impressions.

• Fill your home with photographs of you and your friends doing things you enjoy. Pictures of trips, vacations, and other activities will show visitors different parts of your personality.

• Make your bedroom an inviting space for romantic encounters. Nice sheets and bed coverings needn't be a huge investment, and they'll go a long way toward creating a mood.

• Throw out the futon. A grown man should have a real bed.

• Avoid packaged art. If possible, put original art in your home and avoid posters and other generic prints. Interesting and unusual art doesn't have to be expensive, so use your imagination.

• A coat of paint, curtains, cushions, and other touches can bring a home to life. Even if you don't own your place, treat it as if you do. If you make it a place you like to be, chances are that others will like to be in it, too.

• Buy some house plants. They won't cost you much but they'll instantly add life to any room.

• Don't feel compelled to display glossy coffee-table books and magazines in the living room. The books you choose to read and shelve are a better indicator of your interests and intellect.

• Keep your home looking fresh and clean. Dust and vacuum at least once a week, and make sure the bathroom is a place you won't be embarrassed to have visitors see.

Different ages of sex

Age ain't nothing but a number

Like everything in nature, your sexual response has a life cycle. This cycle is affected by the body's aging process, but it's also closely linked to changes in your emotional development. At different stages in your life, sex will fulfill different physical and psychological needs, and your attitude to sex may vary depending on other areas of your life. Understanding how you develop as a sexual person as you age not only helps you maintain a healthy sex life, it also prepares you for the changing role sex will play in your own life and in your relationships with others as you grow older.

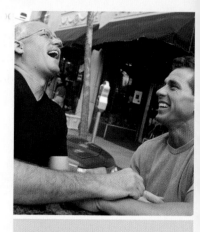

Sex through the years

The stages of sexual development don't always exactly mirror our physical development. In general, however, we can look at sexual development in terms of early years, middle years, and later years. Each stage of our lives has its own characteristics, and the role sex plays in each of them varies—along with all the other changes that aging brings.

We can define the early years as the time when we're first discovering who we are as gay men, and particularly as sexual gay men. For some of us this occurs during the teens

and 20s, but for others it may not occur until the 30s, 40s, or even later. This is particularly true of men who don't come out until later in life.

Regardless of when we begin exploring our sexuality, the early stages of sexual development are usually centered on experimentation. For many men this means having multiple partners

IN MIDDLE AGE we often find our lives have settled into a comfortable pattern that provides a sense of security.

Young at heart

We've all heard the saying, "You're only as young as you feel." Well, you could also say that you're only as sexy as you feel. Many men seem to make the mistake of thinking that just because they're growing older they're growing less sexually attractive. Instead, they should see themselves as possessing sexual experience and skills that men of any age can appreciate.

Does age matter?

Differences in age can definitely affect a relationship, but is there an age gap that's simply too much? Not if both partners recognize that their ages may result in differences in other areas, such as interest in sex, and factors like family, money, and how leisure time is spent. An age difference of 15 years may not seem like much when one partner is 30 and one is 45, for example, but 15 years later when the older partner is entering his 60s, some issues may need to be addressed.

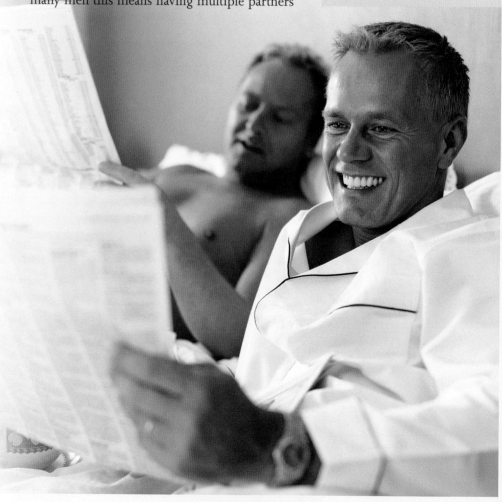

and engaging in sex as often as possible. This stage can be compared to the teen years, when heterosexuals get to date and experiment sexually. Because most gay men don't get to experience this period of development as teenagers, we frequently need to go through it later in life. Finally able to express ourselves openly, we often make up for lost time, sleeping with many different people, perhaps without regard for how this behavior can affect us, or our partners, emotionally.

The middle years

This period of our sexual lives, which may parallel our chronological ages as we move through our 30s and into our 40s and 50s, is generally characterized by looking to settle into relationships. Sexually, we may find that we're no longer interested in experiencing sex with a range of partners and are satisfied with one partner. Rather than being an end unto itself, sex is part of a larger, richer, romantic life. Having become more comfortable with ourselves, sex is less about looking for a source of affirmation and more about sharing ourselves with someone else, whether we're in a monogamous relationship or having sex with multiple partners.

The later years

As we enter our 60s, 70s, and beyond, of course our bodies begin to slow down a bit, and this may affect our sex lives, possibly decreasing the frequency or duration of erections or the intensity of sexual desire. Although many gay men seem to view aging with trepidation about "losing" their looks and the bodies of their youth, the fact is that sexual interest does not necessarily wane just because we're not 35 any longer. Physically, men may maintain active sex lives well into their 80s and beyond.

How we see sex at this stage in our lives depends on a variety of factors, including our physical health and whether we're partnered or

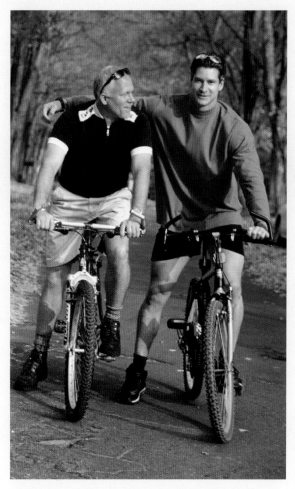

A MIXED-AGE RELATIONSHIP can create opportunities for you and your partner to see the world, and each other, in new and exciting ways—despite the difference in your age.

single. If your sex drive has decreased owing to physical causes, sex may be relatively unimportant to you now. Or perhaps relationships and friendships have assumed much of the role that sex once played. But it's also entirely possible that you're still very much interested in sex, and there's no reason why men in the later stages of life can't enjoy active sex lives.

We're all individuals, so some of us will find that our sex lives follow a natural progression as we age, while others may experience the stages of sexual development either earlier or later than other men, or perhaps out of order altogether. It's important to understand that how we function sexually and how we view our sexuality will change with age. We must also learn to see ourselves as sexual beings at whatever age we are or stage of life we're in.

Changing together

Although the idea of growing older with the same partner is attractive, it's important for couples to realize that changes in their relationship are inevitable as they age.

• Neither of you should be the same at 45 as you were at 25. Give your partner room to grow as a person, and acknowledge that accepting each other's changes can be difficult sometimes.

• If your sexual interests are developing in new or unexpected areas, discuss them with your partner, rather than ignoring or attempting to fulfill them outside of the relationship.

• If your interest in sex varies dramatically from your partner's, consider discussing the issue with a therapist or counselor before it becomes a bigger problem.

• Learn what is exciting about men at all stages of sexual development. This is especially helpful if your partner is older than you are. Imagine what it would be like to be his age and practice seeing yourself as sexually attractive.

• Don't automatically dismiss an older man as unworthy of sexual attention—his knowledge can add emotional, as well as sensual and erotic, depth to your relationship.

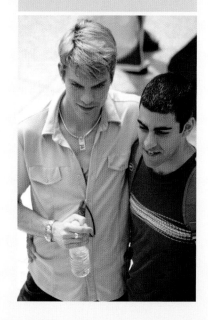

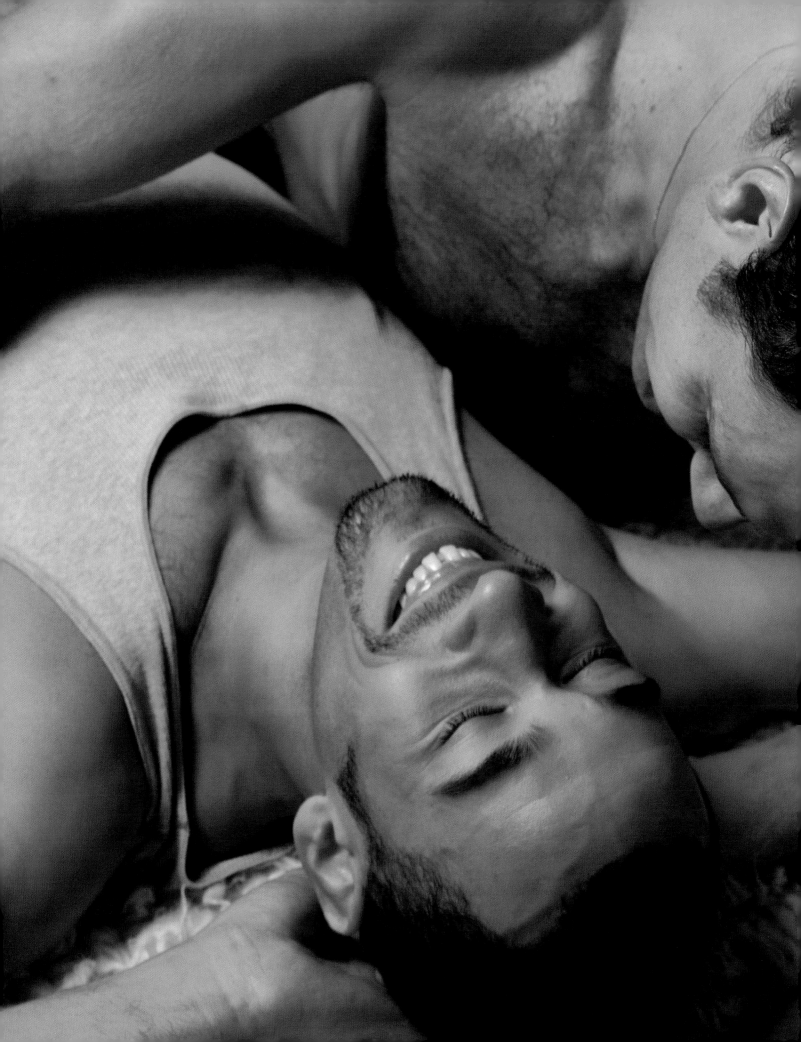

3 You and your partners

Whether you enjoy being single, are searching
for a lover, or already have one, the partners you're
involved with are at the center of your sex life.
Knowing how to find them, and what to do with
them once you have them, means understanding
what you want from your life, and the role sex and
romance play in it.

Singledom vs relationship

Weighing the pros and cons

Single guys have more fun. Guys in couples have more security. Singles are always meeting new people and having new sexual adventures. Couples have established routines that create intimacy. Being single keeps things fresh. Being coupled takes the pressure off. These are just a few of the statements that are often made in the single vs partnered debate. So which is better? Our society tends to uphold the couple as the relationship ideal, but is looking for a partner something every man should have at the top of his to-do list?

In search of someone special

One of the biggest complaints you hear from gay men is that they can't find a boyfriend or partner. Many of us spend a lot of our time thinking about the perfect guy and trying to figure out ways to meet him. Bars and clubs are filled with guys trying to find the man of their dreams, whether it's for one night or for the rest of their lives. So if everyone is looking,

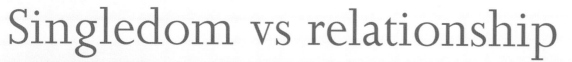

The top 5 reasons to stay single

1 The only person you have to explain yourself to is you.

2 Being with a different guy every time you have sex can make things more exciting.

3 You get the whole bed to yourself when you want it.

4 You can make plans without checking in.

5 You don't get stuck in a routine.

how come so many of us are still single? Is it true that there just aren't enough available men out there? Or is there something else going on, some reason so many of us seem to be looking for something and not finding it? The answer may lie in figuring out whether or not we're really ready to be partnered or if maybe staying single is a better idea for us for the time being. Single life and relationships both have their pros and their cons, and weighing these things against what you want from your life may help you make a decision about what's right for you.

Not just another statistic

What images or feelings come to mind when you think about being single? Do you picture yourself going on dates with lots of different guys, or do you see yourself sitting in front of the television on a Saturday night wishing you had something else to do and someone to do it with? Does the idea of being single make you excited about the possibilities it suggests, or does thinking about yourself being single make you feel depressed and lonely? Each of us has a different concept of what being single means, and examining our feelings about not being partnered can tell us a lot about ourselves and about what we want from our romantic lives.

For some men the idea of being single is exhilarating. They see not being partnered as having the freedom to experience romance and sex with as many different people as they choose to. Without a boyfriend or lover whose needs and feelings have to be considered at every juncture, each new meeting or encounter has the potential for adventure—you're free to decide. And this doesn't apply just to sex. As a single person, you don't have to consult anyone else when making plans or decisions. Your life can be all about you and only you.

THE MOMENT MAY come when you find yourself wondering whether it's time for commitment. Ask yourself whether sharing your life with one other person seems more appealing than having the freedom to do as you wish.

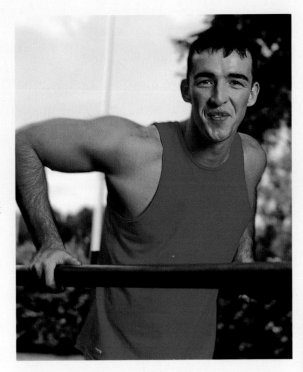

IF HAVING THE freedom to use your spare time in just the way you want appeals, then singledom could be for you, at least for now. If looking for a partner is not top of your list, think of being single as a positive choice.

This freedom is tremendously appealing to some men. Is it to you? Do you like the idea of being able to go where you want to, when you want to, with whom you want to? Does the thought of potentially being able to date lots of different men excite you? Perhaps, for you, being single provides almost limitless opportunities for exploration and fun.

Single, not selfish

Too often we think of single men as people who, for one reason or another, can't find partners. But being single can also be a matter of personal preference. Not everyone wants to be partnered. There are guys who like living their lives solo, who enjoy living alone and spending time with friends, family, and dates when they choose to. Being single doesn't mean being lonely.

So if the upside to singledom is freedom, then what's the downside? For some men dating a lot of different people can be stressful, sending them on an emotional roller coaster. This is particularly true for guys who date multiple

The top 5 reasons to couple up

1 You always have someone to be your date.

2 Being with the same person can make sex more fulfilling over the long run.

3 You have someone to share your life with.

4 You don't have to wonder if he's going to call.

5 Having the romantic part of your life settled frees you up to concentrate on other things.

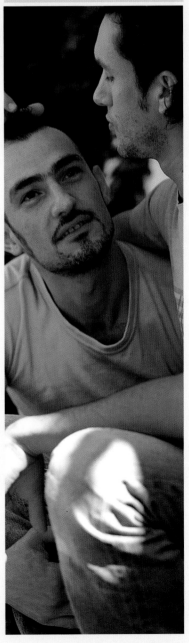

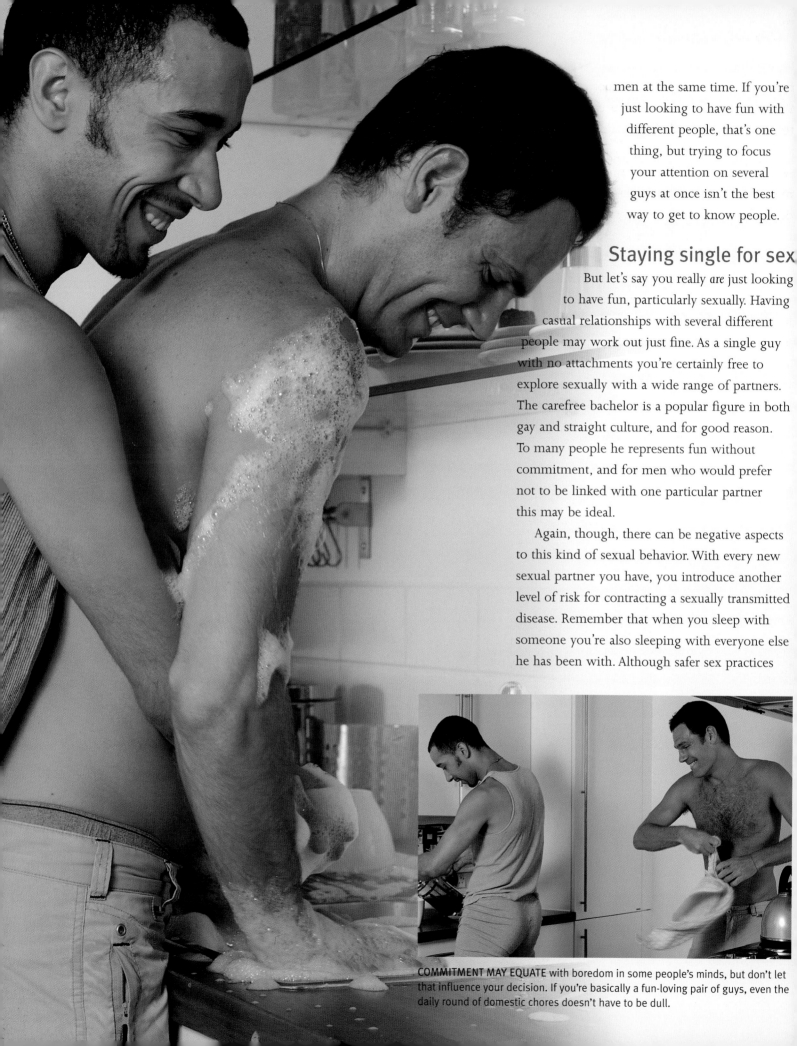

men at the same time. If you're just looking to have fun with different people, that's one thing, but trying to focus your attention on several guys at once isn't the best way to get to know people.

Staying single for sex

But let's say you really *are* just looking to have fun, particularly sexually. Having casual relationships with several different people may work out just fine. As a single guy with no attachments you're certainly free to explore sexually with a wide range of partners. The carefree bachelor is a popular figure in both gay and straight culture, and for good reason. To many people he represents fun without commitment, and for men who would prefer not to be linked with one particular partner this may be ideal.

Again, though, there can be negative aspects to this kind of sexual behavior. With every new sexual partner you have, you introduce another level of risk for contracting a sexually transmitted disease. Remember that when you sleep with someone you're also sleeping with everyone else he has been with. Although safer sex practices

COMMITMENT MAY EQUATE with boredom in some people's minds, but don't let that influence your decision. If you're basically a fun-loving pair of guys, even the daily round of domestic chores doesn't have to be dull.

definitely decrease the risk of exposure to STDs, every sexual encounter has the potential to result in some kind of infection.

Of course, not every single guy has multiple sexual partners—nor is every partnered guy monogamous. Your sexual behavior isn't defined simply by whether you're single or not. But since we are on the subject of sex, let me reiterate the importance of knowing what the potential risks are. If you're a single man who has multiple partners, the fact is that you have a greater likelihood of coming into contact with someone who has an STD, whether it's a simple urinary tract infection or something more serious, such as HIV or hepatitis. So knowing what you may be exposing yourself to is important, as is knowing how to minimize the risk of exposure. See pages 88–91 and 166–169 for more information on types of STDs and practicing safer sex, and educate yourself about what's out there and how to avoid it.

Ultimately, all of us are single at one point or another in our lives, either by choice or due to the break-up of a relationship or death of a partner. We all know that being single sometimes carries with it a harsh and unnecessary stigma. But being alone can be a positive experience, and making the most of it can help us learn a great deal about ourselves, whether we remain single or enter a relationship later on. The important thing is to look at being single as an opportunity for exploration, for growth, or perhaps even for reflection. When you do that, and when you stop seeing being single as something negative, the experience becomes a positive one.

Table for one

For single men, one of the most unsettling situations can be the prospect of eating out alone—even if it does mean having a night off from cooking or takeout food. But dining out alone can actually be a fantastic experience. Instead of worrying about what people will think, how you'll look, and wondering if you'll be seated at a lousy table, act confident and take the opportunity to try different kinds of foods you might not normally eat. The same goes for attending events or going to the movies alone. It can be a lot of fun to experience theater, art, ballet, concerts and other occasions by yourself. Without the distraction of another person, you can focus more fully on the show.

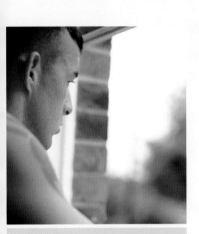

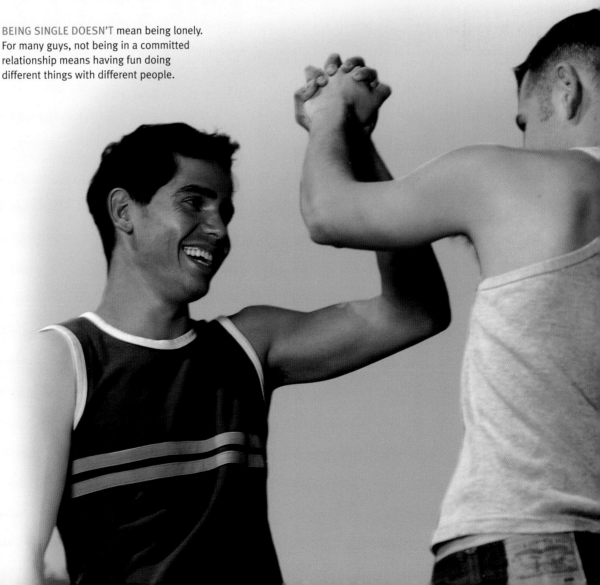

BEING SINGLE DOESN'T mean being lonely. For many guys, not being in a committed relationship means having fun doing different things with different people.

Suddenly single

What happened? Whatever the reason for suddenly finding yourself single, the important thing is to remember that even when you were partnered you were still an individual. Too often, when we are coupled up, we begin to define ourselves, knowingly or not, by our role in that couple, or simply as one half of a couple. Then, when that partnership ceases to exist, we find ourselves without a way to identify ourselves. By remembering that who we are isn't dependent on anyone else, we can maintain a positive outlook on life even if a relationship comes to an end.

Looking at the reality

Despite the fairytale promises of happily ever after, we know that, according to statistics, the majority of relationships end in separation. If this is true, then why do people bother pairing up at all? Why do we voluntarily venture into something that seems almost certain to fail? It doesn't, at first glance, appear to make any logical sense. After all, if relationships are so difficult to maintain, why not stay single?

Part of the problem with this theory lies in the assumption that the end of a relationship can be equated with it being a failure. When, in fact, this is not true at all: What we get out of our relationships, regardless of their duration, is the point of being in them in the first place. Before you discard this notion, think about high-school relationships. The very nature of teenage relationships almost guarantees their failure. Yet high-school hallways are filled with couples, and brokenhearted 14-year-olds will continue to sob over lost loves despite all attempts at reasoning with them.

Wanting to fall in love, and wanting to find someone with whom to share our lives, is a basic human need. No, not all of us want to be partnered and even those of us who do, have widely varying ideas of what relationships are and what part they play in our lives. When it comes to relationships, gay men are at somewhat of a disadvantage right from the start. Unlike our heterosexual counterparts, most of us do not have the adolescent experiences of dating to help us explore our feelings about partnerships. Many of us, in fact, don't have our first real dating experiences until we're in our 20s or even later, when we're out on our own and able to live our lives openly as gay men.

As a result of this, many of us have to play a kind of "catch up," working through, in a very short time, what other people have a decade or more to experience. In addition, we have relatively few role models to base our relationships on. Where heterosexual couples have the relationships of family and society in general as examples of what works and doesn't work, gay men are largely on their own when it comes to defining what their relationships mean.

Why a partnership?

However, there are positive, thriving gay relationships. Many men do choose to partner up and share their lives with someone else. Whereas being single presents us with a potentially unlimited number of romantic and sexual adventures, being partnered might seem to offer exactly the opposite. In reality, what being partnered offers us is the opportunity to get to know someone more and more intimately over a long period of time, a connection that can infuse every part of our lives with a feeling of satisfied wellbeing.

So how do you know if this is something you want for your own life? Start by asking yourself why you want a relationship. Is it because you're looking for someone else to change your life? If so, that's not a great reason to embark on a partnership. If your life needs changing, it has to start with you, not with someone else. It's crucial to realize that the unhappiness you feel with your life situation can't be fixed by finding a boyfriend.

If, however, you're happy with your life, but would like to be able to share it with someone else, then that's a good reason to want to partner up.

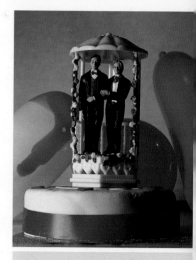

If at first you don't succeed

One of the main reasons why gay men find it hard to believe in the possibility of having a lasting relationship is experiencing the failure of past relationships, either their own or their parents'. It's important to understand that every relationship is different, and that the success or failure of a partnership depends on the two people involved in it. Don't let what happened to someone else, or even what happened in your past, create unreasonable fears and apprehensions. Learn from past experiences and use them to create positive new ones.

If I were the marrying kind

You think you might be ready for a relationship, but how do you know for sure? Before you start looking for that guy to settle down with, ask yourself these questions. Your answers will tell you a lot about whether you're at a point where you can handle the responsibilities of being someone else's partner.

• Are you ready for the possibility of having sex with just one guy for the rest of your life?

• Are you willing to consider someone else's wishes when making plans for vacations?

• Are you ready to deal with someone else's family?

• Are you able to discuss your feelings about issues without getting defensive and/or angry?

• Are you able to compromise, particularly if it means doing something you might not enjoy?

• Are you willing to lose some of your alone time and share living space with another person?

• Are you capable of accepting someone else's faults and admitting to your own?

• Are you happy with your life in general, and do you see being in a relationship as a way to share that life with someone else?

• Are you still holding on to negative feelings or strong emotions from a past relationship?

A relationship is exactly that—a partnership. It's about having someone with whom to share the experiences of your life. Yes, a partner is also someone with whom we make experiences, but a relationship can't *be* your life.

Being in a relationship can, and should, provide you with several important, positive factors in your life, among which you can count companionship, security, and support. Most importantly, a relationship should help you to achieve all the other things that you might want to accomplish in your life. Too often, we think of our relationships as what defines us and our lives. We think of them as though they're the be-all and end-all. But in reality, the relationship itself is not the ultimate goal in life—it is just one of the things that allows you to achieve the life you want to have.

THE BEST DAY OF YOUR LIFE Many congratulations! You've said goodbye to your single days and you're ready to commit to Mr. Right and a lifelong partnership with each other.

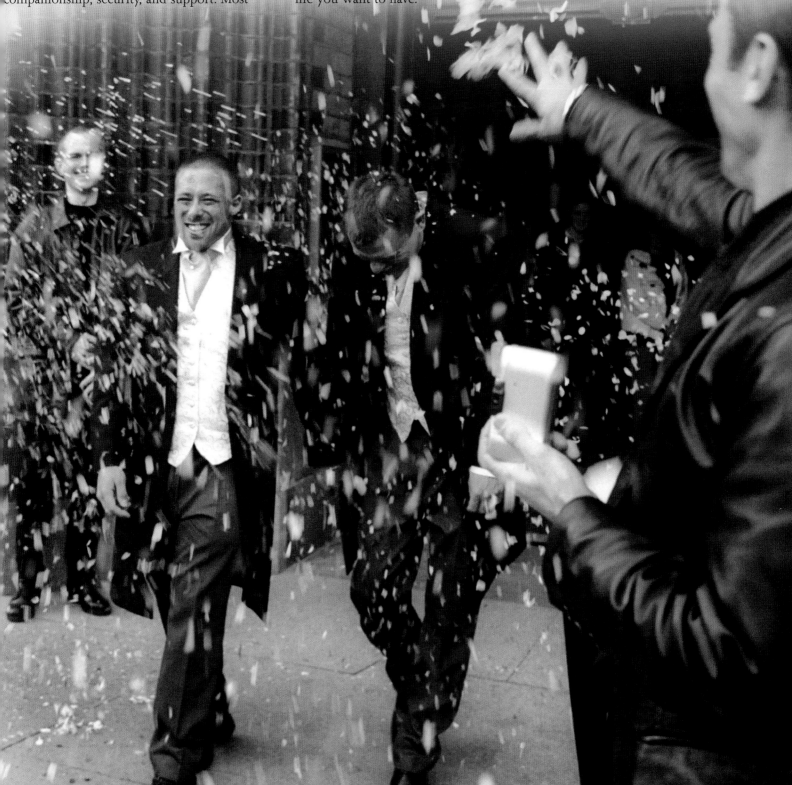

Cruising

Looking for loving

In 1980 the film Cruising, starring Al Pacino and written and directed by William Friedkin, created an indelible image of gay sex: dark, sleazy, furtive, and, ultimately, deadly. For many people, including many gay men, the very word "cruising" came to reflect this world: one filled with desperate men looking for sexual gratification. But what is cruising really about? Put simply, cruising is the playful art of seduction, an erotic adventure in which you explore the various sexual possibilities existing around you. But like all sexual activity, cruising means different things to different people.

Places to go, people to see

Have you ever walked by a guy on the street, caught each other's eye, exchanged lingering glances, and felt a little jolt of sexual desire? That's cruising. Have you ever found yourself taking a stroll through a park to see who you might run into there, or driven your car to a parking lot where other men are parked, and sat there waiting to see who might show up? That's cruising too.

Cruising comes in many forms, from simply sitting at an outdoor café and watching the men go by to actively seeking out sexual encounters in a men's room, on a beach, in a park, or in

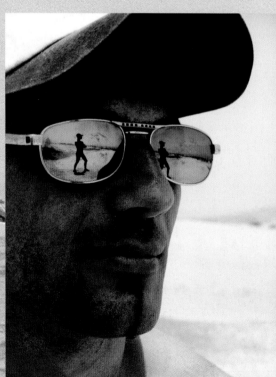
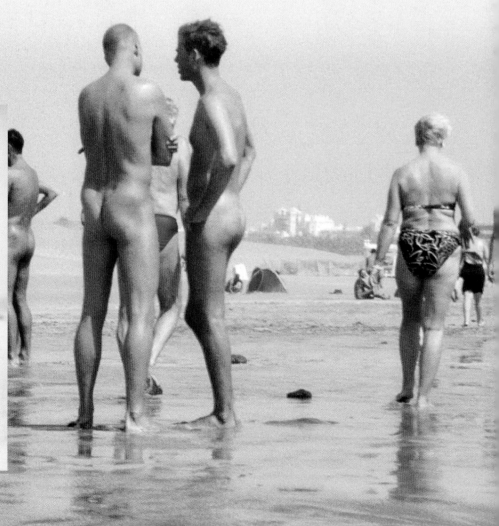

USE EYE CONTACT to indicate interest in someone you're cruising. A direct, lingering look into his eyes (with or without dark glasses) will let him know that you're offering more than just a glance.

Cruise control

Although cruising can be a part of a healthy sex life, becoming obsessive about it or relying on it as your primary outlet of sexual expression can be symptomatic of sexual compulsion. It's easy to become addicted to the thrill provided by having sexual encounters with strangers, especially if you prefer quick sex without the emotional interaction. The problem is that a sex life comprised exclusively of these encounters not only exposes you to greater risk for contracting sexually transmitted diseases, it also prevents you from establishing more substantive relationships. If you find yourself looking for sexual release solely through anonymous encounters, consider looking for help from a mental health professional or from a group specializing in sexual addiction to find out why. It could be that you're using anonymous sex as a way to avoid interpersonal relationships.

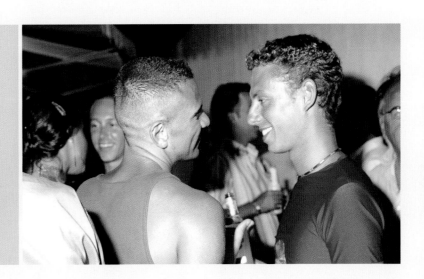

some other place where men go to find each other. In a sense, cruising is like hunting, and in this case it's for sex.

Cruising certainly isn't limited to gay men, although we do seem to have perfected the art more than our heterosexual counterparts have. And not all gay men engage in cruising. Like any other sexual activity, whether you do so or not depends on what you like and what you're looking for. Even though cruising is an activity some gay men excel at, it doesn't mean that all of us know how to do it. In fact, some of us don't know the first thing about it, and are totally oblivious even when we're the focus of a blatantly obvious cruise.

So it's good to know the basics of this timeless art, both in the event that you want to attempt it yourself and, more importantly, in case some hottie is trying to get your attention.

NUDE BEACHES, with their carefree atmosphere and emphasis on displaying your body to passersby, provide an excellent atmosphere for looking for a little fun in the sun.

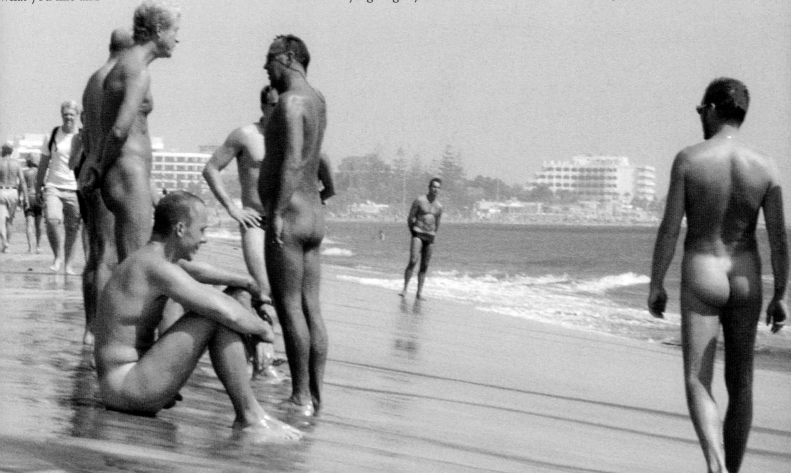

Safe at any speed

While simply cruising a hot guy on the street is usually harmless enough, other types of cruising—particularly any activity involving looking for sexual encounters in remote locations or public areas—is potentially dangerous. In addition to possibly being illegal (make sure you know your local laws), you may also be exposing yourself to the threat of violence. Know the risks of any activity you engage in, and know how to protect yourself in the event of trouble.

After all, if you haven't learned the rules and you don't know how the game is played, you're never going to score.

The most important aspect of cruising, as in any sexual activity, is communication. The difference with cruising is that often this communication is subtler than it is in most other interactions. For example, if you smile at a man on the subway and he smiles back, it's possible he's just being friendly. On the other hand, perhaps he's saying more than just "good afternoon" or "hello." Perhaps he's letting you know he finds you attractive.

How can I be certain?

How do you know for sure? Well, you've got a couple of options. The one you use depends on several things, mostly the situation and your level of adventurousness. Let's take the guy on the subway. First, you could try meeting his gaze again and seeing if he holds your look. If he does, chances are he'd welcome a conversation.

In that case, you could make your way over, or perhaps even get off at his stop and strike up a conversation there.

But let's say you're not on a subway. You're on the street. You pass a handsome man and he gives you a look. Before you can even return it, he's probably walked by you, right? In that case you stop, turn, and see if he's doing the same thing. If he's interested, the chances are that he is also turning around for another look—in which case you have an opportunity to say hello and take things from there.

Perhaps he isn't standing there looking at you though. Maybe he's stopped and is looking in a shop window instead, or checking out the menu outside a restaurant. So what do you do then? The same thing. Give him a chance to catch your eye again, in case he's stopped in order to give you time to figure out that he's interested. Better yet, go over to the window or the menu he's looking at and look with him. If he's interested, you can bet he'll find something to say to you.

A typical cruising scenario

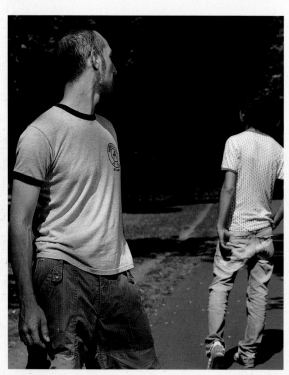

THE CLASSIC CRUISING SCENARIO involves counting to three after passing a guy you're interested in, then turning to see if he's looking back at you.

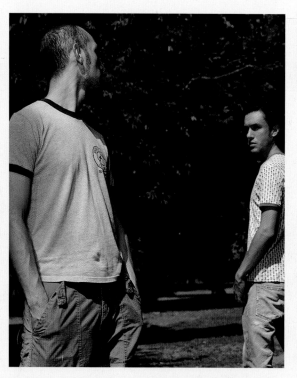

IF HE RETURNS your cruise, hold his gaze and give him a smile or a nod to let him know you mean business and to encourage conversation.

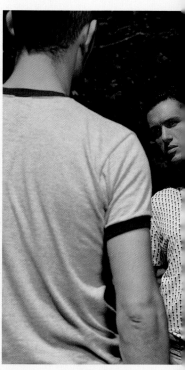

ONCE YOU'VE GOT his attention, approach him and strike up a conversation to gauge his interest.

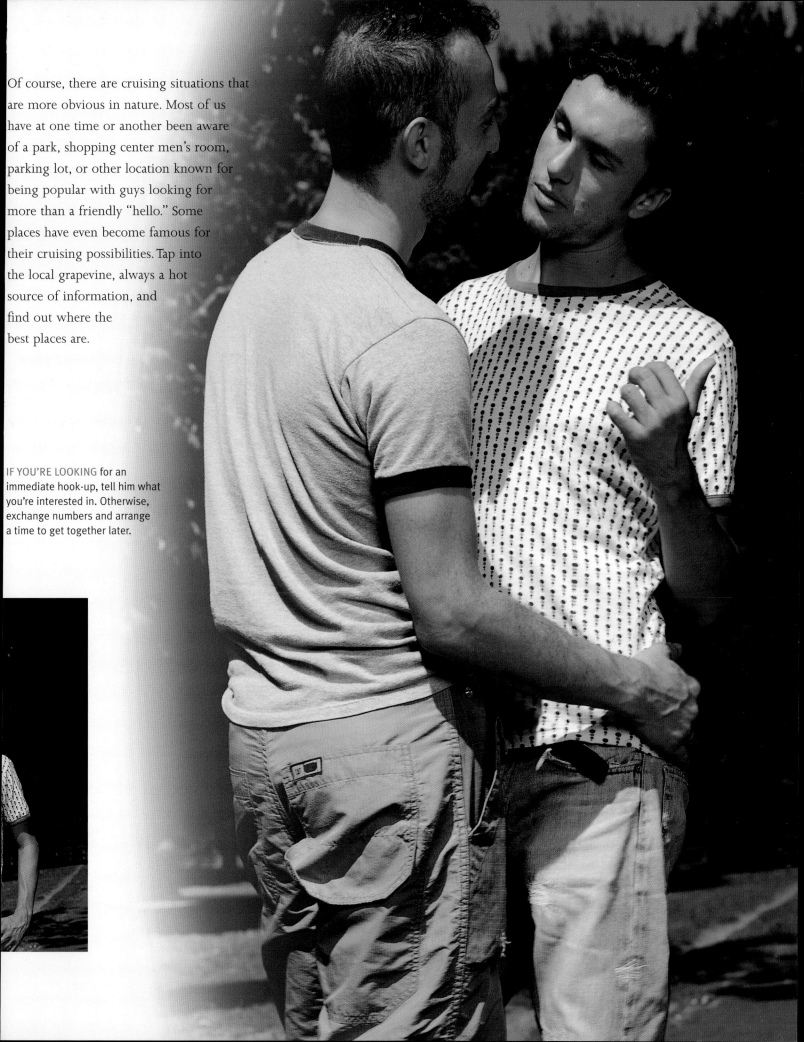

Of course, there are cruising situations that are more obvious in nature. Most of us have at one time or another been aware of a park, shopping center men's room, parking lot, or other location known for being popular with guys looking for more than a friendly "hello." Some places have even become famous for their cruising possibilities. Tap into the local grapevine, always a hot source of information, and find out where the best places are.

IF YOU'RE LOOKING for an immediate hook-up, tell him what you're interested in. Otherwise, exchange numbers and arrange a time to get together later.

The ground rules

What are the rules in popular cruising grounds? Basically, they're all about communication. Sometimes this is really obvious, but at other times the situation might be a little more ambiguous—say, when you and a potential partner have to decide if you're after the same thing. Walking through a park and having someone motion for you to come meet him behind a tree is pretty

obvious, but if the guy beside you at the urinal at the ballpark sneaks a glance at what's in your hand, it might not be more than simple curiosity. If you're unsure what someone is suggesting, go slowly. If the guy at the urinal beside

MAKING THE MOST of the opportunities the men's room can offer is just a question of making sure your message is clearly understood.

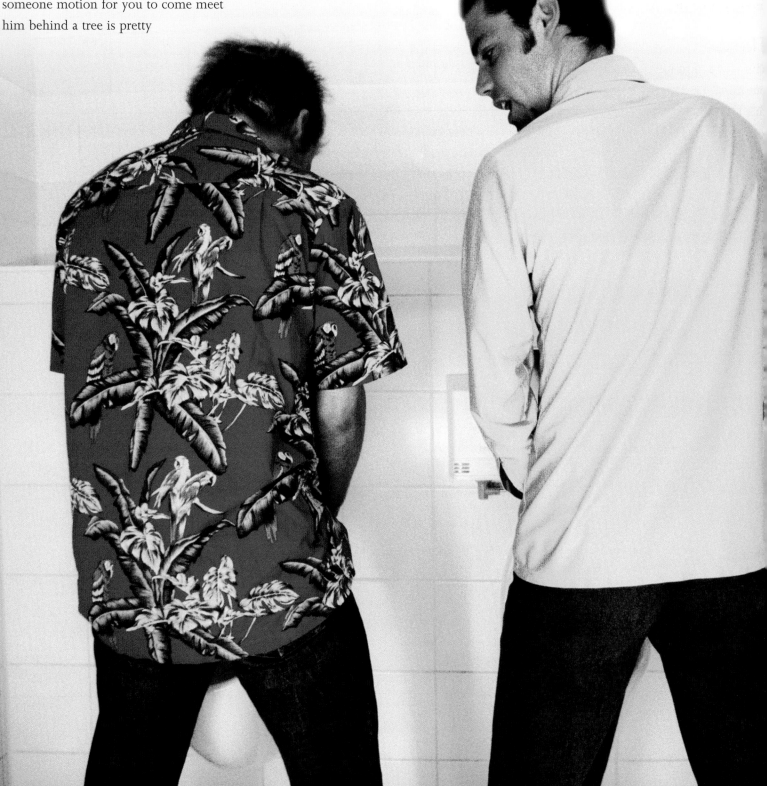

ou finishes but doesn't zip up and leave, you now he might be looking for some action. f the man parked next to you at the rest stop eeps looking over and nodding, he's probably ot there just for a cup of coffee.

There are various techniques for letting a guy know you're interested and they work n different cruising situations. Two of the most popular are "the look" and "the foot tap."

The look

This is the most basic of all cruising techniques, but it may be the hardest to perfect. There's a ine line between simply flashing or returning a friendly smile and imbuing that look with a ittle something extra that holds the other guy's attention. The secret is in the eyes. When you make eye contact with someone who interests you, hold the look for longer than usual. Most people look away after only a second. If you can manage to hold contact for three to five seconds, he'll know you're being more than just friendly.

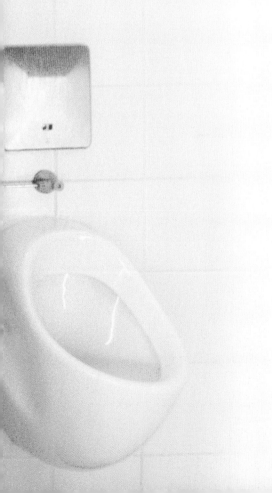

"The look" works in situations as diverse as scoping out the crowd at a bar, passing a man on the street, or cruising a department store. Men, in general, don't look one another in the eyes unless they mean business. So if someone unexpectedly gets your attention and doesn't look away, take it as a hint that he might like to spend some more time with you.

The foot tap

Originating in the stalls of men's rooms, this worldwide signal is still most effective in that environment. If the fellow in the stall beside yours slides his foot closer and closer and starts tapping the toe, you can be pretty sure he's looking for a buddy. But the technique works—with slight variations—in other situations too. Let's say you think the guy seated next to you on the airplane is worth checking out. Try pressing your knee against his. Sure, he might think you're just a space hog, but if he presses back and leaves his knee there, you might be in for some in-flight entertainment.

Whatever the cruising situation is, it all comes down to letting your potential partner know what you want and what you're available for. If you send mixed signals, chances are you'll just end up confusing each other. If you keep meeting someone's gaze, for example, be sure you're really ready to talk to him, in case he decides to start a conversation. If you're not interested in him, stop looking at him. Similarly, if a guy whose attention you're trying to attract never smiles back at you, don't assume he's playing hard to get. Just accept that he's probably not interested and move on.

So remember, cruising is ultimately a game: you're trying as hard as you can to get someone to notice you, or someone is trying their best to get you to notice him. Approach cruising as a source of fun—whether it's while walking your dog around the block or lounging on a nude beach in the altogether—and it will be a pleasant, and potentially rewarding, experience.

What are you saying?

Cruising has a language all of its own, and knowing what particular signals mean—and how to use them yourself—is important. If you give a guy mixed or unclear signals, he's going to get confused, or even frustrated, and move on. So be sure that your body language is conveying the right message. Here are some tips:

• If you're not interested, make it clear. Don't return his looks or other signals. If necessary, walk away or move to another spot.

• Remember that even though an encounter may be anonymous, you're dealing with a real person. Don't be hurtful or cruel to anyone, and if you need to say no, do it as politely as possible.

• When cruising somewhere new, watch the other guys to see if there are any particular rules or signals that are used.

• Keep in mind that sex in public places is often against the law. If you play in public, know what you can and cannot get away with, and what your legal rights are.

• Don't spend too much time waiting for him to make the first move. If you both keep waiting for a sign, nothing will ever happen.

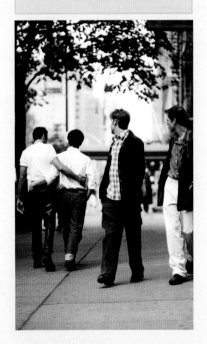

Finding a lover

When and where to look for a partner

I remember waking up with the first guy I ever slept with and thinking, "He's my boyfriend and we're going to be together forever." Okay, so I was wrong. He didn't become my boyfriend. But I was young, and I think many of us, when we start dating and having sex, make finding a lover the all-important goal of everything we do. We worry about where to find him, how to get him, and what to do once we have him. Some of us get so obsessed with finding The One that we make ourselves crazy, convinced that our lives won't be perfect until we're paired up once and for all.

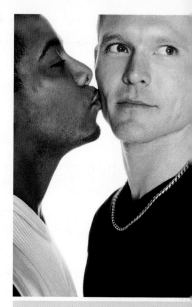

Life's no fairytale

There are so many things wrong with this attitude it's difficult to know where to start. The number one truth about relationships is that finding a lover won't make you happy unless you're already happy. You can shake your head all you want to, but it's true. And I'll tell you why—because being happy comes from liking yourself as a person, and from being fulfilled by what you're doing with your life. Another person cannot make you happy; he can only make you happier. Another person cannot fix what you don't like about yourself or about your life; he can only share the life you already have. If that life isn't enough without him, it's not going to be enough with him.

I can see all of you hopeless romantics out there wailing in despair. Get over it. The notion of Prince Charming coming along and taking you away from it all is an illusion. If you're thinking that everything will be great once you find a man to love and to love you back,

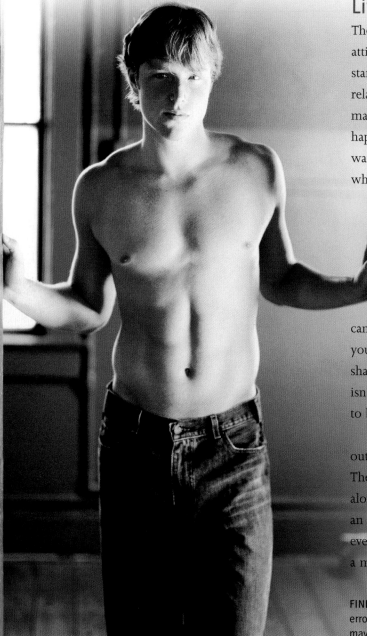

FINDING MR. RIGHT can be a matter of trial and error, so take your time. No matter how much you may want someone to be The One, don't hurt yourself by jumping into a relationship too soon.

The one for you

One of the best things about dating is the first rush that comes with meeting someone new, when everything seems magical and perfect. But those first few days, weeks, and even months, are usually not accurate predictors of what a long-term romance with someone is going to be like.

Caught up in the thrill of being with someone new, it can be difficult to tell whether an attraction to a guy is based on simple physical attraction or on something a little deeper than that. And if the sexual chemistry is on, it can make it easy to ignore signs that the relationship might not be everything we think—or hope—it is.

So how do you know? When evaluating a romance for its long-term potential, ask yourself what you find attractive about the relationship, and particularly about the guy at the center of it. If most of your answers have to do with how good things are in bed, or romantic notions rather than reality, take a little more time to get to know your man before deciding he's the love of your life.

It may take a couple of months or even a year or so to be absolutely certain he's your ideal guy, but this is the time to experiment and have a little fun while you find out.

you're selling yourself—and love—short. Love is not something to use as a magic wand or a cure-all. It is something that you share with someone else, and you can't do that effectively when you're depending on that love to make you the person you dream of being.

First, be happy

Think about it this way: Two halves do indeed make a whole, but only if those two halves are already complete unto themselves. And no, this isn't some weird Zen koan. It's reality. Unless you and your partner are already happy as individuals, you're not going to be happy as a couple. And if you're not happy as an individual when you start looking for a lover, you're going to end up settling for some guy who you think is going to make everything okay. And I guarantee you he won't make everything okay; he'll just make you even more unhappy.

So before you even think about finding a lover, take a look at your life as a single person. Are you happy? Do you like what you're doing? Do you have friends and interests that are an important part of your life? Is a lover something you would like to have and not something you think you *have* to have? If so, then you're ready to start looking.

If, however, you aren't particularly happy with your life, if you spend a lot of time thinking about how things would be so great if only you had a man to be with, then you've got some work to do. Take some time to think about what it is about your life you're not satisfied with. Maybe it's your job, your apartment, or your appearance. Try to pinpoint what it is you're dissatisfied with, then look for ways to remedy the problem. Once you've gotten yourself to

a place where you're satisfied with who you are and where you're going, put finding a lover back on your to-do list.

When you're ready

Now let's say you're happy with your life and you're ready to find someone to share it with. What do you do? Well, you can either sit back and just wish and hope or you can be proactive and do something. This means making a couple of decisions. First of all, what kind of guy are you interested in meeting? If you know what you want, it will make things a lot easier. So make a list. Sit down and think of some of the characteristics you'd like a partner to have. You can certainly include physical things, but traits that have to do with personality, beliefs, and attitudes are more important. This list is meant to be a rough set of guidelines, so don't be too rigid about your requirements: You don't want to pass up guys who would be great partners. But writing a list is a good place to start.

Fantasy or reality?

When choosing potential partners, be sure you're going after what you really need in your life, and not some sexy but inappropriate fantasy. Just because you find a particular look or a certain image appealing, it doesn't mean that every man who has it is a good partner for you.

Don't be taken in by appearances, and make sure you get to know the real man underneath the surface before you decide a guy is the one for you. Being attracted to someone doesn't mean he's going to give you what you need emotionally, and you may find that the fantasy you've created doesn't hold up so well in the real world.

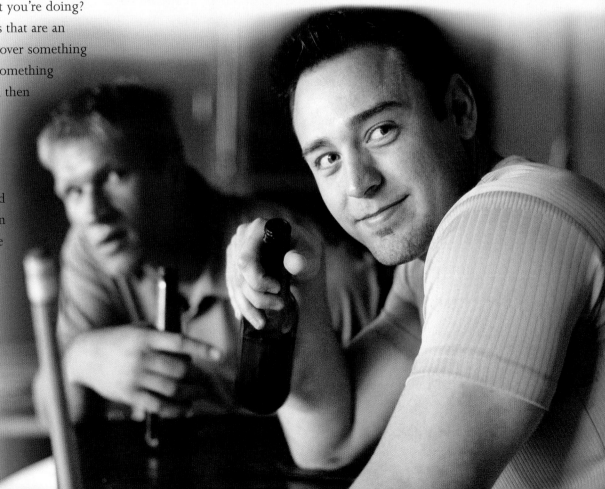

HUNTING IN PAIRS won't necessarily double your chances of capturing a prospective lover, but your network of friends is a guaranteed way in which to get out there and meet more men.

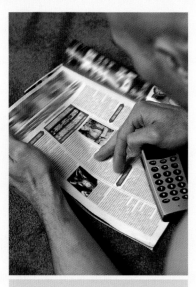

Classified info

Looking for a lover using classified ads can be a great way to meet other guys. Classifieds aren't solely the domain of newspapers—think how much farther your ad will travel via the internet. Learning a little classified shorthand will help, as will keeping your wits about you; some people are *very* creative writers. The fun—and addictive—part is replying to other guys' ads.

Where to look

Once you've got your list completed, look at it and see if you can find clues there to help you decide where to start looking for a potential partner. Is physical activity a big part of your life? Maybe your lover is waiting for you in one of the many sports clubs available to gay men. Does your ideal guy have a passion for politics? If so, volunteering for a political candidate or a political cause might bring the two of you together.

There are many, many places other than bars or clubs to meet men, so expand your horizons. Social clubs catering to every interest from line dancing to leather, cooking to discussing books and movies, can be excellent venues for interacting with other men. You can even meet guys at churches, synagogues, and other religious meeting places. By becoming more involved in things that you enjoy, you're likely to meet other men who also enjoy those things.

Don't forget about your friends, either. They know lots of people you don't, and one of their friends might be someone you find absolutely wonderful. I met my partner when

a mutual friend invited us both to a movie. So if you're interested in meeting new guys, put the word out. And if a lot of your friends are looking for partners, consider having parties where you each invite a few friends outside your immediate circle. Then you can all have a chance to meet new guys in a setting you're comfortable with.

The next thing to do is take a reality check. Meeting new people is exciting, and making a sexual and romantic connection is particularly exciting. Sometimes it's so exciting that we forget that first impressions (and sometimes second and third impressions) are not always accurate. We're all on our best behavior when we meet someone new, and it's easy to think that the great new guy you're interested in is absolutely perfect.

He's not. None of us is. But often it takes a while before people figure that out. So when you do meet that man who seems to have everything you want, don't be so wrapped up in the excitement and the fantasy of him that you ignore potential issues. This doesn't mean you should go looking for problems, it just means you need to keep a clear head about things.

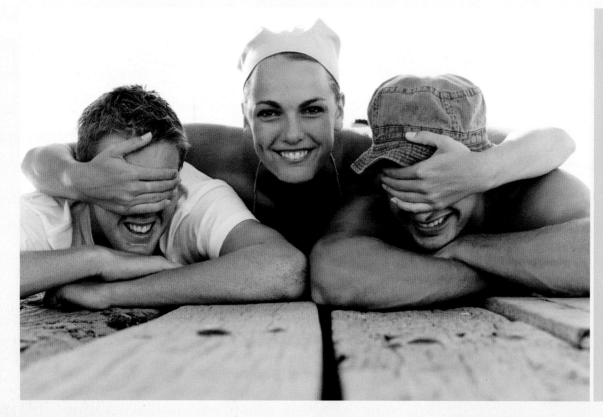

I have this friend

Setting friends up with each other is always a gamble, but it can also produce some surprising results. Just keep these suggestions in mind before playing matchmaker.

• Don't tell them you're setting them up. Arrange for them to meet under neutral circumstances.

• If they do get together, let things proceed naturally. Stand back and see how they progress as a couple.

• Don't share private details of either friend's past with the other. Let them get to know each other at their own pace.

• If the relationship doesn't last, don't get in the middle of any resulting ugliness. Try to remain neutral and discourage any badmouthing of either party.

Enjoy your relationship on a day-by-day basis and really get to know one another before you make any decision about where things are going.

Take your time

One of the biggest mistakes gay men make is going for the first guy who seems to fit the bill. You don't have to do that. In fact, I insist that you don't. Very few guys are going to be good partners for you. Although the idea of falling wildly in love right away is appealing to many of us, acting impulsively more often results in unsatisfying, and even disastrous, relationships than it does in lifelong togetherness. In an ideal world, a lover is someone who you will be spending a very long time with. Although we all want different things in a partner, at the heart of any relationship should be a man you enjoy sharing your life with. Don't mistake simple sexual attraction for something lasting, and don't be in such a rush to settle down that you settle for something less than what you want and need in your life.

WHAT'S THE RUSH? The longer you spend getting to know someone the more comfortable you'll be in each other's company. You've got the rest of your lives ahead of you, so don't put yourselves under pressure by committing to one another early on.

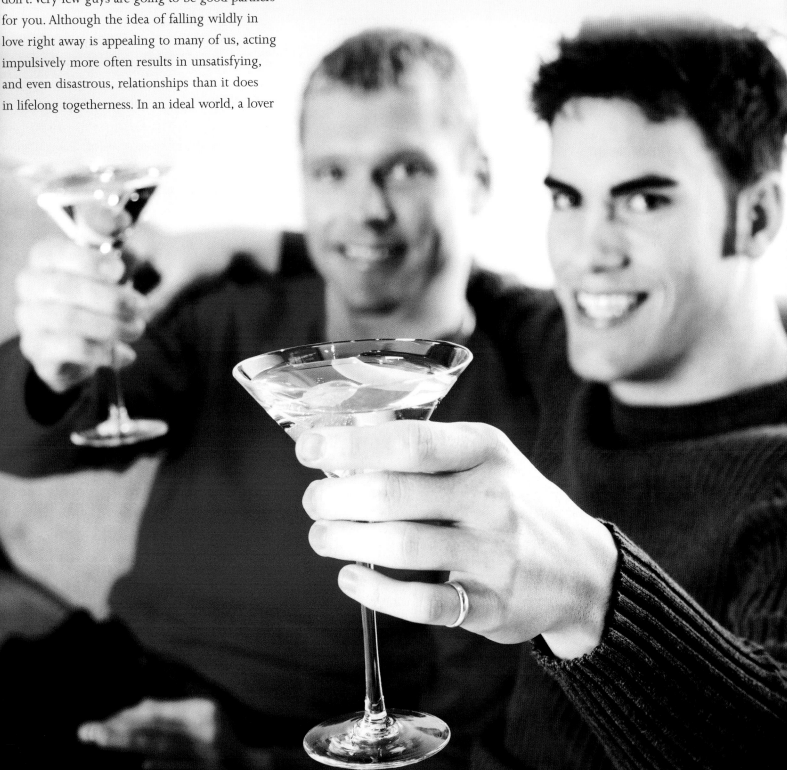

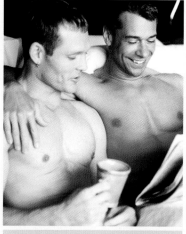

Places to go

Where to rendezvous

Back in the dark ages, the only place where gay men could meet was a bar. Okay, so it's only about 35 years since the dark ages ended and in some places bars are still the primary venue for gay men looking to meet other men for sex, friendship, or both. But most cities offer multiple options for gay people to get together and even in small towns, with a little looking, you can find ways to meet up with other men. So whether the bar scene is for you or not, stop complaining that there are no ways to meet people. Take a look.

Paper talk

When you are vacationing together or doing business alone in an unfamiliar city, the best way to find out about the local bars and clubs is to pick up a copy of the local gay newspaper. Many bars cater to a particular clientele, and knowing whether a nightspot is a leather-and-Levi's hangout or a dance club will help you to decide where your time is best spent.

Happy hours

Gay bars and clubs are still one of the primary meeting places for gay men simply because many guys feel comfortable in these settings. In general, you can assume that everyone there is gay and is hoping to meet someone. Knowing that, guys feel free to cruise, to talk to one another, and perhaps to initiate sexual activity. But are bars and clubs ideal meeting places for gay men? They can be good options, particularly if your choice is limited by where you live. But establishments like this can also pose some problems. For one thing, by their very nature, bars and clubs encourage alcohol usage. Although drinking might remove some inhibitions and help you to relax, too much alcohol may well impair your judgment and cause you to do things you might not otherwise do.

In addition to the booze, the loud, frantic atmosphere of most bars isn't exactly conducive to getting to know someone. So, if you're looking for more than just a quick hook-up or a fun night out with friends, you might want to skip places with pounding music and dim lighting and look elsewhere.

Breaking through the bars

Clubs and bars aren't the only options for meeting people, and in fact it's best if you look beyond them for ways to find new friends and partners. Our lives are—or should be—about more than drinking, dancing, and hanging out, hoping we'll run into someone worth getting to know better. By exploring things that interest

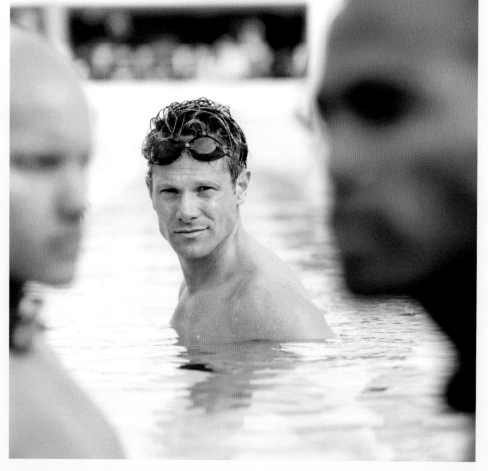

THE MORE EFFORT you put into meeting guys the greater your chances of success. Get out into the real world and discover the best that the gay lifestyle has to offer.

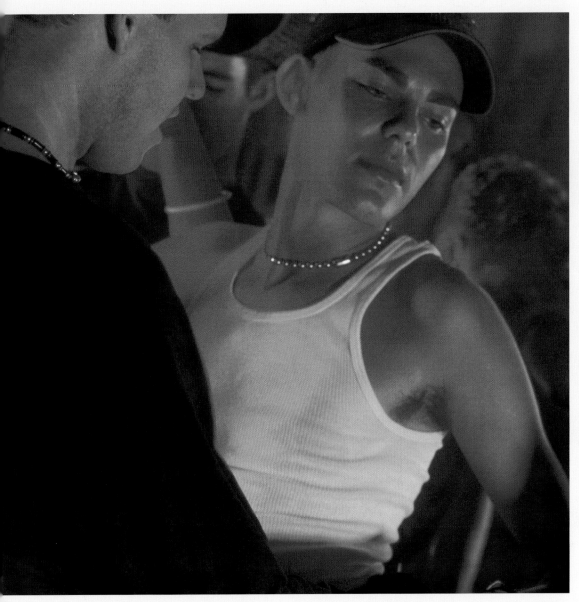

Keep an eye out

Sometimes when we're having a good time at a club, the excitement we feel can lead us to do things we might not normally do. One way in which to protect yourself from engaging in potentially embarrassing or unhealthy activity is to make a deal with the friends you go out with to watch out for one another. If one of you looks like he's about to do something stupid, the others can step in and intervene.

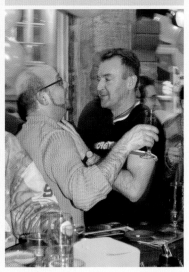

FOR MANY GAY guys bars and clubs represent the most logical place to meet other men, but they aren't necessarily the best places to find long-term partners.

you, you stand a much better chance of meeting someone who shares both your interests and your outlook. And by getting out of the bars and into the world, you help yourself become a more well-rounded person, a person other men will be attracted to.

Think about the kind of guy you want to meet. Now think about where you're likely to bump into him. Chances are, you want him to share at least some of your interests. So doesn't it make sense that the best way of finding that type of guy is to get involved with the things you like to do? After all, if you're looking

for sushi you don't go to a steak house, and if you're into baseball you don't go to the ballet hoping to catch a game. It's just common sense.

Get organized

Make a list of the things you like to do. Now make a list of the things you're looking for in a guy. Are there items both lists have in common? If so, start from there. If you like sports and you want to meet someone else who enjoys them, join a gay softball team, soccer league, or scuba-diving club. They all exist, so check them out and see if you meet someone you like. Even if you don't, you'll be doing something you want to do, and will be making new friends (who, by the way, may know just the guy for you).

Lend a hand

One of the most rewarding things you can do in life is volunteer. The gay community offers many opportunities, and while you're at it you just might meet someone.

• AIDS hospices and support organizations, gay youth groups, political causes, community centers, choruses, and gay pride festivals all rely on the help of volunteers to keep running.

• Gay sports teams and social groups often have volunteer boards and are always looking for help.

• Choose something that you're truly interested in and make a commitment to it. Don't just go once or twice and leave because no one catches your eye. Persist!

You've only got to go out and socialize—it really is one of those rare and fabulous situations known as a win-win.

Is your spirituality important to you, and do you want a partner who also finds it an important aspect of his life? There are groups for gay Buddhists, Catholics, pagans, Muslims, Jews, Episcopalians, Hindus, and every other belief system. Go to a service or meeting. Get involved with a church or temple. Imagine your mother's face when you tell her you met a great guy at the synagogue or Midsummer ritual.

If religion isn't your thing, maybe politics is. All kinds of gay political groups exist out there, all of them looking for volunteers to help spread the word. Similarly, there are many different gay groups centered around occupations, from firefighters to lawyers, doctors to dock workers, teachers to journalists. Take a look around and see what's out there. Not only do these kinds of groups provide chances for romance, they're also great networking opportunities.

What's your hobby?

When it comes to hobbies, the possibilities are almost endless. Into motorcycles? There are gay riding clubs. Riding and roping? Try out the gay rodeo association. Join a gay book discussion group, a chorus, a running club—anything you think is interesting and fun probably has an organization of other people who also enjoy it.

And what if there isn't a group? Then start one. Get going with a few friends who share your interests—poker, say, or skiing—and have them invite other people. Put an ad in the local gay paper. Spread the word about your gay hockey league, dinner club, or hiking group and see who responds. You'll be surprised what happens when you put the word out.

By now you get the idea—live your life and let the opportunities for meeting people present themselves. Too often we focus so hard on the meeting people part that we forget about everything else. But meeting someone can't

be the primary goal of an activity. It should be a rewarding by-product of living a productive, well-rounded, and satisfying life.

Sexual encounters—or more?

If you're just looking for sex, fine. Go to a sex club, visit internet chat rooms, cruise areas known for sexual activity. But if you're looking for more than that, create an interesting life for yourself before you look for someone to share it with. Finding someone to be with won't give you the life you want. You have to have that life first. Then the kind of guy you're after will come into your life because you'll be putting yourself in places and situations where he's likely to be.

So start thinking about life beyond the bars. Instead of heading out for a Friday night of drinking and hoping you'll get lucky, go to a film festival or a play. Rather than spending your time leaning against the wall at a club waiting for someone to talk to you, sign up for a gay cruise or travel adventure. Take a two-step class or a sign-language course. Take a gay literature or Italian class at the local university or learn how to cook. Do something just for the fun of it and you might just be surprised at how much you get out of it.

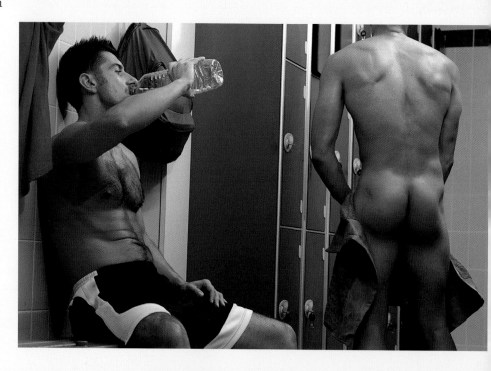

Is it cool to throw a dinner party?

Of course! Because most of us have such busy lives, it's rare that we actually have people over for dinner. Junk food, takeout, and meals-on-the-go are ruining the art of socializing. But the old-fashioned dinner party can be an excellent way to introduce your friends to one another and to meet friends of theirs you might not know.

Try organizing regular dinner parties—say once a month—for your friends. It doesn't have to be formal; the point is just to get everyone together in a casual setting where they can relax and let the wine and conversation flow. Have everyone invite one other person who you don't know. At worst, you'll meet some interesting new people and, with a little bit of luck, you could meet someone you want to share dessert with.

USE YOUR HOBBIES to create opportunities for meeting men. Playing for a gay sports team, for instance, can be an excellent way to meet potential partners who share your interests.

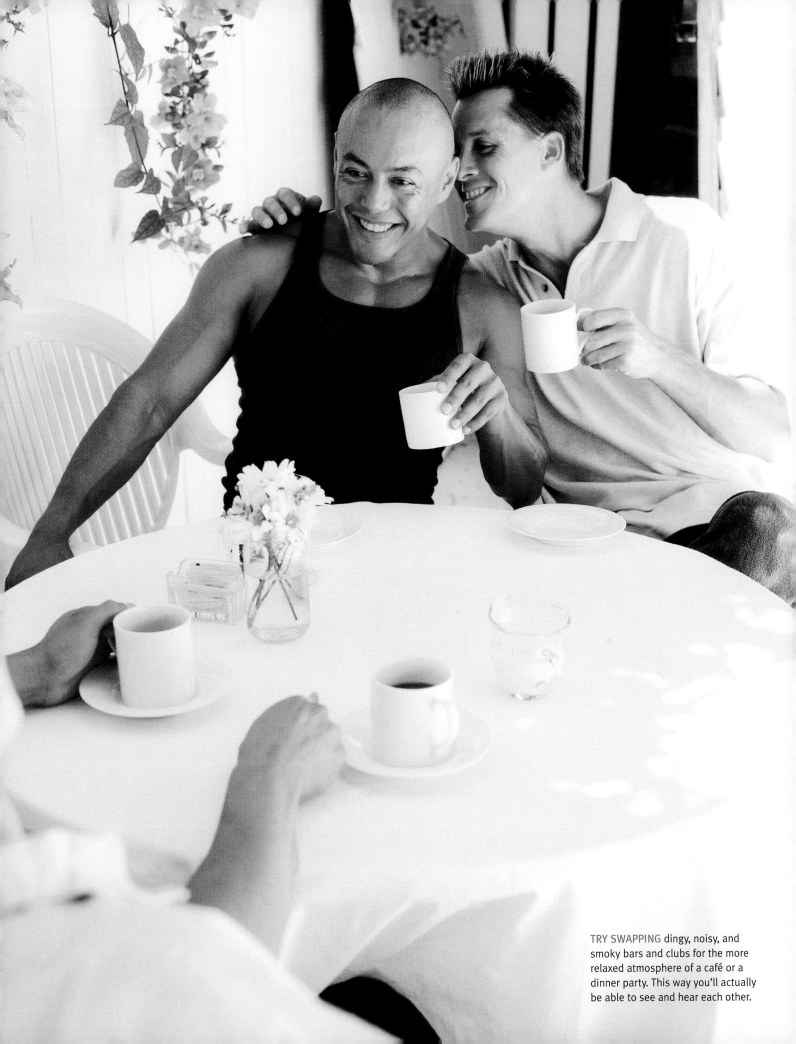

TRY SWAPPING dingy, noisy, and smoky bars and clubs for the more relaxed atmosphere of a café or a dinner party. This way you'll actually be able to see and hear each other.

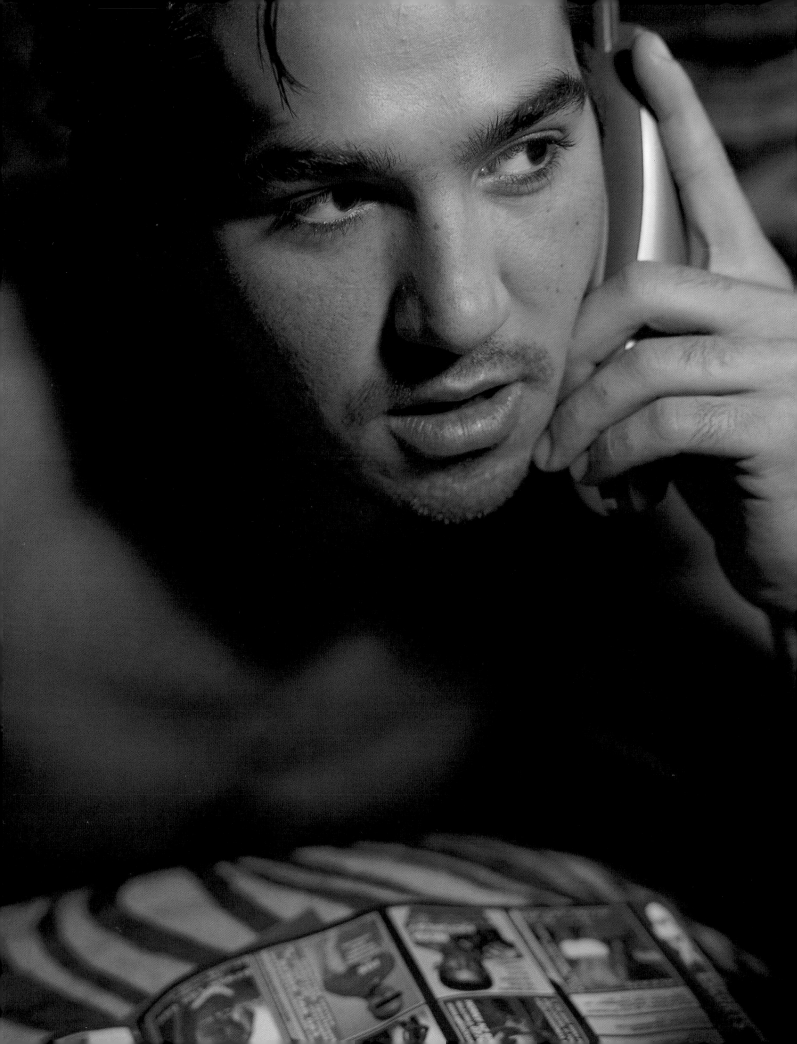

Phone and internet sex

Making connections

In this age of technology, it's not surprising that sex has moved from the bedroom to the computer screen. Internet chat rooms, websites, and webcams are all tools you can use to look for sex, learn about sex, and even have sex. The good old-fashioned telephone, too, provides fantastic opportunities for finding and having sex, whether with a current partner or with someone new. With so many different outlets available to you, knowing how to make the most of them will make your time online or on the phone much more fun and rewarding.

Cyber safety

Using the internet and phone lines to find guys for real sex is fine, but there are some rules you need to follow to make sure you're playing as safely as you can. Before you agree to meet up with that hottie you've been flirting with, keep the following in mind.

• Any encounter with someone you don't know has the potential for danger. If possible, meet him on neutral territory (a coffee shop, say) before doing anything else.

• If you just can't wait to get it on, at least insist that you talk by phone before you arrange a get-together. Never give him your address without speaking to him first. If he's not willing to give you his number, forget it.

• Never use fake photos to entice someone into playing with you. Sending images of porn stars or guys you find online, even if they really do look like you, is not cool.

• Remember that not everyone is who they say they are. If he sounds too good to be true, he just might be. Have realistic expectations, and if he turns out to be someone you're not interested in, politely end the date or encounter.

EVEN WHEN ENGAGING in virtual sex with someone you know, it's fun to play around.

Close encounters

There are many reasons for utilizing the internet and the phone for sexual purposes. It may be that you live in an area where other gay men are few and far between, and online chat rooms and phone lines are a way to meet people for sex. Or you may be involved with someone who doesn't live locally (or a partner who travels frequently), and online encounters or phone sessions allow you to enjoy each another sexually when you're not together physically. And then some men simply enjoy the experience of living out their fantasies verbally, or via computer screens.

Be creative

Whatever your reasons, there are things you can do to ensure hot encounters. Remember, with only voice or written stimulation to work with (unless you're using a webcam to send visuals), you and your partner need to rely on your imaginations and your ability to create a scene and mood.

Simply telling someone that you want to go down on him might be enough to get him off, but it isn't very sexy. Create some atmosphere instead. Tell him how the back room of the bar smells, or what the hayloft of the barn looks like. Describe how feeling his hands on your body is making you want to suck him off.

The best part of phone and internet sex is that you can look like you want to look and do what you want to do. This is about fantasy, so let your imagination run wild. Even if you would never lick someone's boots in real life, you can do it because this is your fantasy and anything goes. Unless you really plan to meet each other in person, feel free to describe yourself as a 6' 4" construction worker with a 10-inch penis, when you're really a 5' 8" accountant with an average endowment. Create scenarios and see what happens. Be the bad cop and the suspect he's interrogating. The more you involve your imagination, the more surprised you'll be at where it takes you.

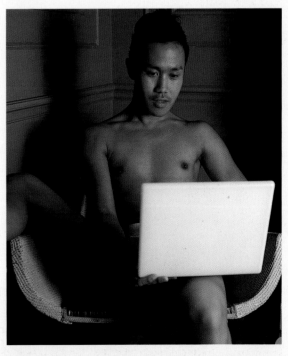

THE INTERNET IS an exciting world, where your fantasies can be played out and satisfied in countless ways.

Casual sex

A lifestyle decision

I've always liked the phrase "casual sex" because it implies that there's "formal sex," rather like how many companies have "casual Fridays," when workers wear jeans and T-shirts instead of business attire. When I hear someone mention casual sex I can't help but picture guys who are really laid back, perhaps sort of indifferent to the whole thing or simply relieved that they can get away with not taking it as seriously as they would if they were having formal sex. So what is casual sex? Well, that depends on your definition, so let's look at the different possibilities.

Playing by the rules

If you have a regular partner with whom you have casual sex, it's important that you establish ground rules and stick to them. For example, agree that you will always wear condoms when engaging in certain activities. If you both know what the other expects, there's less room for misunderstandings or surprises later on.

At some point you and this partner may decide to make the transition to something more serious. It's important that you discuss what the new boundaries of your relationship will be. Will either of you continue to have sex with other people? If so, are there certain activities you'll reserve only for one another? Are you going to see each other a certain number of times a week? Get it out in the open.

Free and single

In general, casual sex refers to sexual activity that involves no defined emotional component. It can refer to one-night stands, anonymous encounters, or even sex with a friend or fuck buddy. It's casual, not because you don't take it seriously, but because neither you nor your partner expects anything from the other apart from the sex itself.

Casual sex is in some ways the fast food of sex—easy, tasty, and with no particular lasting value. This doesn't mean it's not fun, or even a positive experience. It just is what it is, and like that burger and fries you grab on the run, it can be something you might buy from time to time or an indulgence you enjoy a little too much.

Some people believe that all gay men are interested in is casual sex or that all gay men engage in casual sex. This isn't true, of course, but casual sex often does play a role in our development as gay men and in our sexual lives.

How casual is casual?

When we first come out and begin exploring our lives as gay men, with a whole world of opportunity open to us, it's natural to want to experience and enjoy as much as possible. For many men that means going to bed with different people and trying different things. There's nothing wrong with this, of course, but it is important to keep a few things in mind and actively think about what you are doing. After all, you are responsible for yourself.

ONE-NIGHT STANDS, chance encounters, or sex with friends or fuck buddies ... casual sex opens up a whole new world of exciting opportunities to the single guy.

Even the most casual sex affects us in some way. Making love with someone, even if we never know his name or see him again, brings up feelings and emotions, even if those feelings have nothing to do with the particular man we've slept with. Perhaps being with him makes us realize that what we really want is a more lasting relationship—a relationship with commitment and ties.

Maybe something that happens during sex brings up fears or anxieties we have about our bodies or our attractiveness. Possibly the encounter leaves us feeling a little awkward, ashamed, or even depressed. These responses have little to do with the person we've had sex with, but they are very real feelings that can last long after he's gone home. If this happens, it's important to examine your

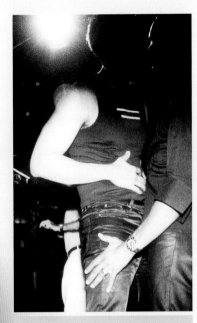

How careful do I need to be?

Just because you're casual about sex doesn't mean you should be casual about your health. In fact, the more partners you have the more you're exposing yourself to the possibility of contracting a sexually transmitted disease. Be sure you know how to prevent and recognize the symptoms of STDs. It's important not only to keep yourself healthy but also to be mindful of how you might be affecting the health of your partners.

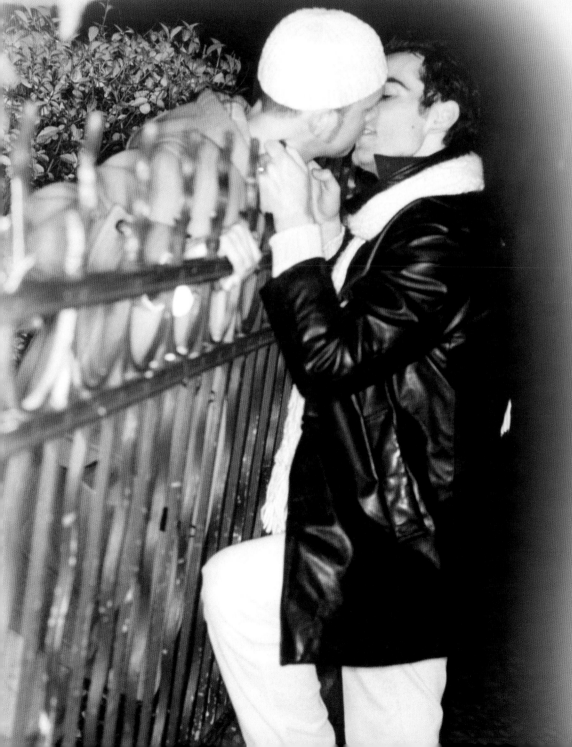

AND YOUR NAME IS? The anonymity of relationships centered on casual sex can add to the mystique and intensity of these kind of partnerships.

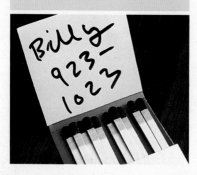

feelings and try to understand why you're having them. Is it perhaps because you were always made to feel bad about how you look, or maybe because a previous lover teased you about some physical characteristic?

Are you someone who, consciously or not, believes that if someone has sex with you he wants to have a relationship with you? These kinds of feelings can affect how you respond to having casual sex and should be considered when deciding what your personal rules are.

More than just sex?

It's easy to turn a casual sexual experience into more than it is, particularly when you're having your first, real, adult sexual encounters. While the other guy may just have wanted to get off, you might start thinking that he's the one you're supposed to be with. You may imbue the experience with far more emotional content than it actually warrants, building it up and up until the fantasy bursts, and you're left saddened over the failure of something that never really existed.

Be realistic about casual sex. If you meet a guy in a bar and go home with him, that's really all you're doing. Sure, it may eventually develop into more if both of you are interested in that, but at first it's just sex. You don't know enough about each other for it to be any more than that, so don't turn it into something it's not.

At the same time, don't treat it like it's just an accident. It's okay to want to have sex with someone. It's okay to go home with someone and have wild, hot sex even though all you know is his first name (if that). But it's only okay as long as you accept it for what it is. It's when you start attaching all those other fears, hopes, dreams, and shame to it that sex becomes something unhealthy.

Nothing more, nothing less

Now don't get me wrong. I'm not saying you should run around hopping into bed with everyone who offers. What I'm saying is that

exploring or expressing your sexuality through casual sex doesn't make you a bad person and doesn't mean you're not capable of having more lasting relationships. Strings of one-night stands are no more satisfying or healthy for you than a diet of potato chips and soda. But every so often a candy bar hits the spot, and as long as we include it as part of a well-balanced life, it's okay.

The trick, so to speak, of enjoying casual sex is to remember that these encounters are about enjoying yourself and about expressing yourself as a sexual person. They're no more and no less. They may become more, but initially they're solely about getting off with someone else. If you always keep that in mind, you're far less likely to turn them into opportunities for emotional drama.

Fuck buddies and other partners

In addition to one-night stands, casual sex can also involve sex partners you see on a regular but not exclusive basis. These could be guys you have no other connection to apart from your sexual encounters. They can also be people who are friends but who you also engage in sex with—fuck buddies. Possibly they're even exes you still enjoy having sex with. The point is, the sex you have with them isn't part of an existing, larger, romantic relationship. While these kinds of relationships can work successfully, they also present some challenges.

Contrary to what we're often taught or expected to believe, it *is* possible to have fulfilling sexual encounters that have nothing to do with love, at least not with the kind of love we think about when we talk about romantic relationships. Casual sex with relative strangers can be more adventurous, more experimental, and more breathtaking than the sex enjoyed by those in longer-term pairings. And sometimes sex with people who we relate to primarily as friends, or even with people we only relate to sexually, can be just as wonderful and positive as sex with someone we're partnered with.

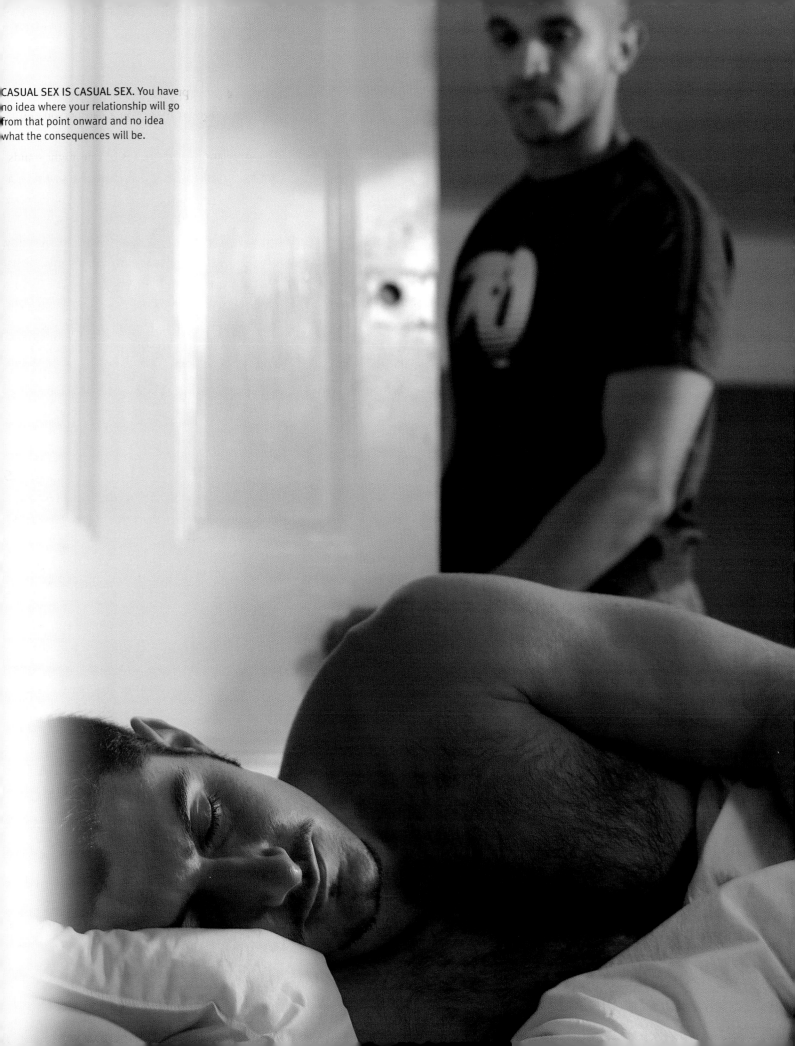

CASUAL SEX IS CASUAL SEX. You have no idea where your relationship will go from that point onward and no idea what the consequences will be.

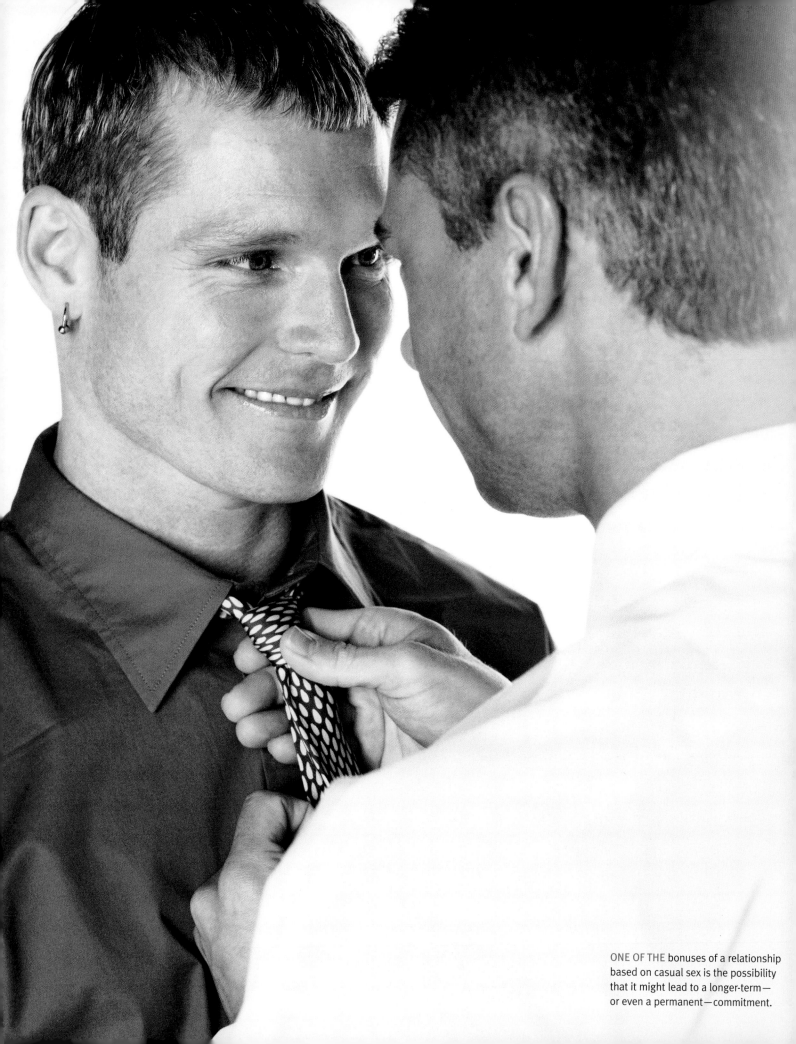

ONE OF THE bonuses of a relationship based on casual sex is the possibility that it might lead to a longer-term—or even a permanent—commitment.

Can I put the "ex" back in my sex?

We break up with people for a lot of reasons, not all of them negative. And sometimes even after the breakup we still find ourselves sexually attracted to our ex. It's not unusual for people to continue to have sex with an ex even when the relationship is over. And this is okay, provided both people understand that it's just about the sex and nothing more than that.

If you want to fool around with an ex, just keep in mind that it's very easy to slip back into relationship mode. Remind yourself why the relationship didn't last and, if necessary, remind your ex too. If you can't have sex without it churning up your past, call it quits, no matter how hot his hairy chest makes you or how much he likes it when you go down on him.

Just one of the guys

It's true, having respect for a sexual partner is important. And having affection for a partner adds another dimension to sex. But you don't have to be in love with someone for sex with him to be satisfying. It's entirely possible to have one or more people who fulfill a sexual role in our lives, whether they fill other roles or not.

Some men, either purposefully or without really planning to, create a group of people with whom they can engage in sexual activity without becoming romantically attached. For example, they might get together regularly with a group of guys they feel comfortable with for masturbation or other sex acts. Or they have just one other person whom they like to get off with from time to time, a guy who they find sexually appealing but who is not someone they want a deeper relationship with.

These people may be friends, acquaintances, or even exes. Whoever they are, the point is that they provide a safe way to express your sexuality.

You feel comfortable with these people, and sex with them is fun because it comes with no accompanying baggage. (Okay, there might be just the tiniest bit of baggage with your exes.) Sex with them is easy because you know what to expect and you know it isn't going to turn into some big drama.

As with all sexual activity, the key to making these casual relationships work is communication. With anyone you have sex with (but particularly with exes) it's crucial that you discuss what each of you expects from the situation, and what you're willing and not willing to contribute to it. If it's just sex, make that very clear. You don't want having sex with someone to mess up any other relationship you have with him.

As casual as you like

It's important to remember, too, that casual relationships shouldn't be used as replacements for more intimate relationships. It's possible you simply aren't interested in anything more than sexual relationships, and that's okay if it's what you really want to happen. But, in general, casual situations are ones we get into either before we decide to settle down or when we're between relationships. Sometimes they exist while we're in relationships as well, but that's another story. The important thing is to know what role you want these types of partners and encounters to play in your life.

Whether there's a guy you call every couple of months to come over and ride you hard, a group of buddies you meet with for some JO action, or an ex whose oral skills you just can't say no to, casual sexual relationships can play an important part in a healthy sex life. But they work only when everyone involved understands what the rules are, and when you understand what the encounters do and do not mean. As long as you are clear about this, casual sex can be a very positive experience.

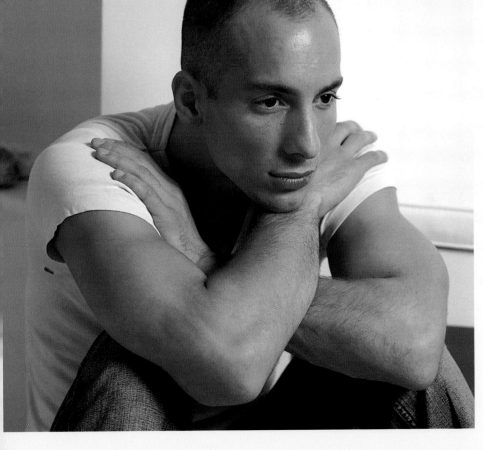

FOR ALL THE highs and exhilarating times having casual sex can bring, be prepared to accept that it isn't unusual on some occasions to be left feeling frustrated or lonely.

Relationships and couples

Sharing your life

Being part of a relationship is something many (but not all) men look for. We form relationships for many different reasons, some of them emotional and some of them practical, but whatever our reason, understanding how relationships work and the role that sex plays is an important part of creating successful partnerships, and developing a fulfilling sex life with a lover. And since the place sex holds in a relationship often changes as the relationship progresses, it's good to examine the different issues that may arise as time passes.

TIME SPENT TOGETHER doing routine things, such as making dinner or taking care of household chores, helps couples develop a sense of togetherness that makes both partners feel comfortable and secure in the relationship.

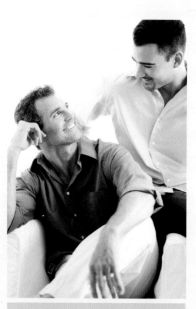

Friends and lovers

Every good relationship needs to be a good friendship as well. Your partner should be someone you trust to be there for you, and who you are willing to support in turn. This doesn't mean you have to do everything together all the time. In fact, you should have friendships outside your relationship to help maintain a healthy balance in your life. Otherwise you risk putting too much pressure on your relationship to fulfill all the needs in your life. Be sure you and your lover both have interests and friendships outside your relationship, and encourage spending time pursuing your individual hobbies and pastimes.

Sex isn't everything

At the heart of every relationship, should be a fundamental desire to share your life with another person. It's a wonderful experience for partners to be able to watch and help each other grow into the people you are both meant to become. A partner should be more than just someone you live with simply because it's convenient, more than just someone you find physically attractive, more than just someone you have great sex with. A partner should be someone who makes your life richer on all sorts of different levels.

Sex is a natural expression of relationships. Again, sex shouldn't be the thing that you base your relationship on because, as great as sex is, it's not something that should define who you are and what your life is about. Rather, it should be something that you enjoy doing with a partner simply because it reflects and expresses other, more important, aspects of your relationship.

When we have sex with someone, we are, both literally and metaphorically, exposing ourselves to him. When sex occurs within a wider relationship, it often mirrors other things about that relationship that are important to us. Perhaps we're more relaxed or open when we're making love with a partner whom we trust not to hurt us or to laugh at something we might like to do sexually. We're certainly less vulnerable.

We feel more in control. Maybe through sex roles we can act out other roles that are important to our relationships.

There are many ways in which sex within a partnership can deepen that relationship. Sex can heal us, or inspire us, or reveal other sides of our personalities. And that's where knowing someone intimately helps make sex even better. When you understand what your partner likes and how he thinks, you have an excellent foundation for making sex incredibly fulfilling for both of you.

Can't get out of bed

When a relationship first begins, it often seems that you're having sex practically all the time. The newness of your partner, and the thrill that comes from finding someone attractive, and having him find you attractive, combine to create a potent effect. Making love seems like the most amazing thing you could ever do, and you're sure that you'll never tire of having sex with this man. And maybe you won't. But for most of us, that sexual fire eventually burns down. This doesn't mean we've lost our attraction for our partner. On the contrary; it means that the frenzy of sexual excitement that we felt initially has grown and deepened into something even more fulfilling.

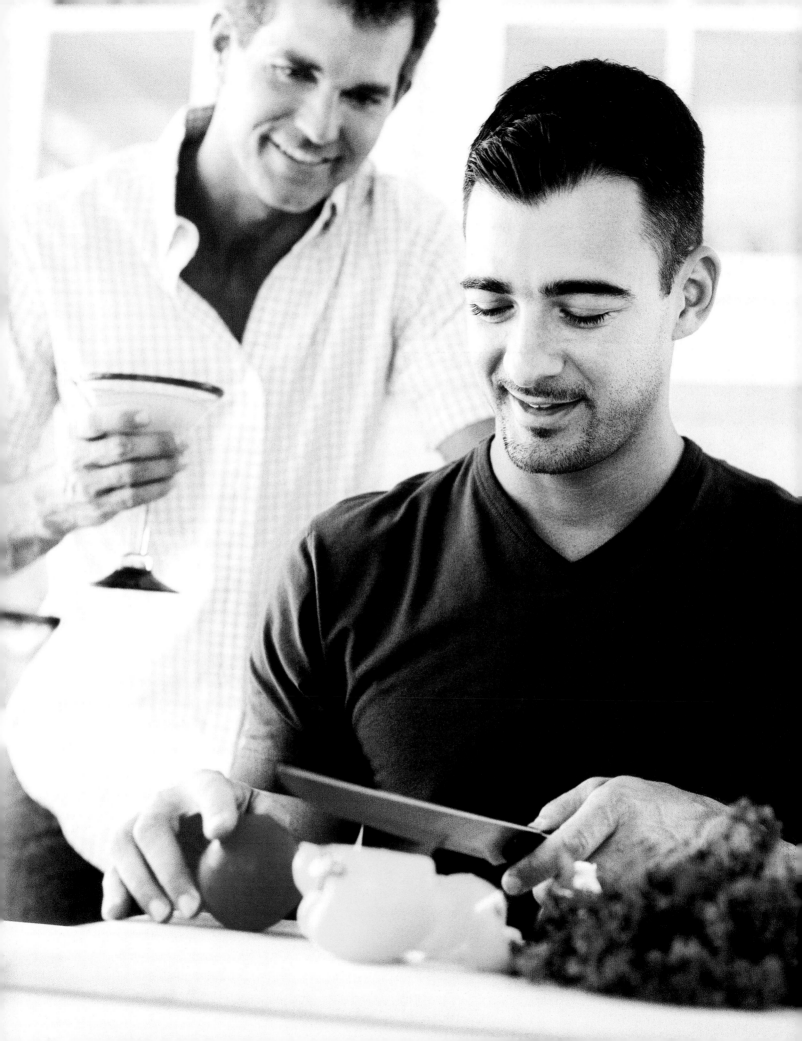

Frequently in new relationships we use having sex as a way to confirm our interest in this new person. Because we don't really know each other all that well, we need something with which we can measure our compatibility. If he finds us sexually attractive and we find him attractive, we reason, then things must be on the right track. Then, as our comfortableness with the relationship grows and our need to reassure ourselves that everything is okay diminishes, sex takes on a more relaxed role.

The problem is that as a relationship goes on you can't (and shouldn't) apply the same standards that you used to evaluate the relationship when it began. We have sex for many different reasons. How often you have sex with a partner should not be a gauge of the health of your relationship. Certainly a noticeable lack of sex is reason for concern, but much more important is the quality of the sex that you do have. It doesn't matter if you have sex every day, every week, or every

Sex or love?

Don't mistake hot sex for love. Being sexually compatible with someone doesn't necessarily mean he'll make a good partner. Take time to get to know the guy, in and out of bed, before taking things further. If you try to build a relationship based solely on sexual chemistry, chances are your romance will crash and burn as soon as the fireworks die.

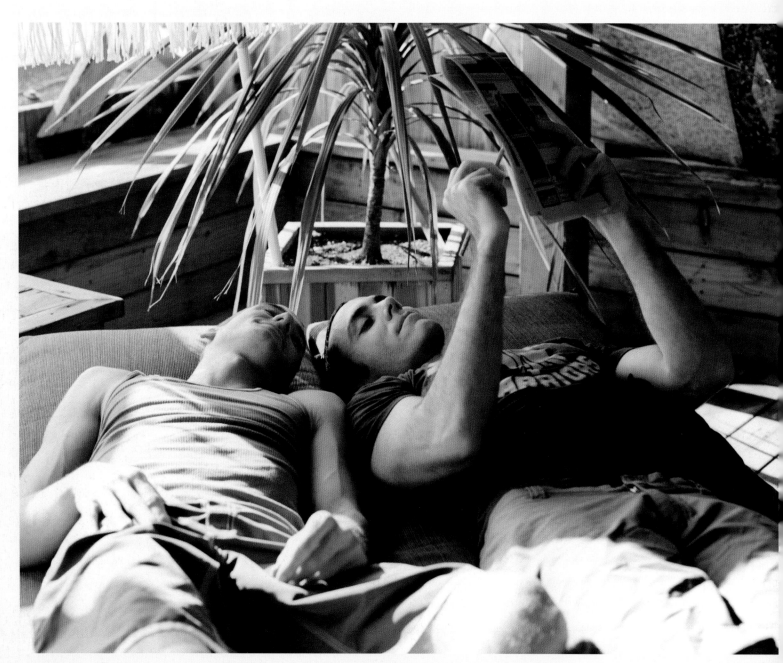

AS YOUR RELATIONSHIP develops and deepens, you may find that you want to take the next step, sharing living space. When this time comes, discuss what you both expect from living together before you move in.

month as long as the sex you're having with your lover is fulfilling to both of you. If it isn't, then you have a problem.

Happy talk

What's important to remember is that you and your partner are individuals, and you won't necessarily have the same sexual interests and needs, particularly as your relationship goes on and you grow as people. So within your relationship it's important to create an approach to lovemaking that allows you both to express and yourselves and enjoy yourselves. And the key to accomplishing this—as it is to so many things in life—is good communication.

Yes, this means you have to talk about sex. It's funny how we can be intimate with someone in so many ways but still be afraid to talk to him about sex. But if you want to develop a healthy sexual relationship with your partner, you do have to talk about it, and not only when there's a problem. You have to be able to talk about it even when things are going great. You need to be able to tell your guy what you like about him sexually, and what you want to do with him.

When you can have this kind of honest dialogue about sex, you're going to prevent 99 percent of the problems that arise from sex. If you know that you can discuss absolutely anything with your partner, and if he knows he can bring up any subject with you, you're not going to hide things or let small issues grow into larger ones. Also, you're going to create an atmosphere in which sex can only become better and better.

Relationships don't (or shouldn't) remain static. They change over time as each partner changes individually and as each lover learns more about the other. Although, for many people, it's tempting to want things to remain the same forever, this really isn't a healthy attitude. Change may sometimes be

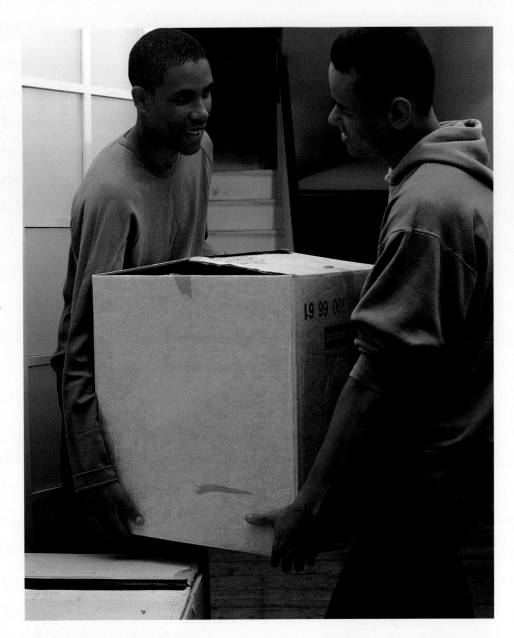

MOVING IN WITH a partner is an important declaration of your commitment to each other, symbolizing your desire to build a life together. It's an occasion where you are openly displaying your long-term intentions.

frightening, but when you understand that it is actually a reflection of growth, then it appears less threatening.

In the early stages of a relationship sex may be the primary focus because it's the most intimate experience that you have with this new person. With time, however, how you relate sexually very often changes and, as you feel more comfortable with each other, sex may become a less significant aspect of your life together.

Not tonight

We aren't always on the same sexual schedule as our partners. Sometimes stress, health issues, or other concerns mean you won't want to have sex when he does, and vice versa. Don't have sex just because one of you wants to. Either compromise (perhaps by having the horny partner jerk off while the other watches or helps out) or decide to put sex off until a time when you're both up for it. Whatever you do, don't feel guilty, or make your partner feel guilty, for not being in the mood.

Fear of change

Many of us don't like change. It's threatening. We feel more comfortable knowing that things will always be the same, that the garbage will be collected on a Tuesday, that we'll walk the dog at 7am, that we'll cook dinner every other night. This is especially true when it comes to our relationships. Knowing that our partners will always be the men we fell in love with takes away a lot of the insecurities we have about being ourselves, and about being part of a couple.

But change happens. As we age we learn more about ourselves. We develop new interests, and the things we need from our lives don't always stay the same. It's important to accept these changes, even when they're frightening or when they mean making decisions about our relationships. Generally a fear of change is really a fear that a partner will leave us or that a relationship will end. We see changes in ourselves or our partners as signs that something must be wrong. These changes are a natural part of growing as individuals, and a healthy relationship can easily withstand them. If you feel stressed or apprehensive about changes in your life, talk to your partner. If you can't, or if you need an objective perspective, speak to a counselor.

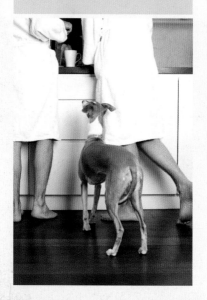

Spicing things up

Similarly, some men find it easier to be less inhibited with someone they don't know well. At first, it may be easy for sex with a new partner to be wild and hot because there are no expectations of what things *should* be like. Because our partners don't really know us well at this stage of a relationship, we can be whomever and whatever we want to be sexually. Then, ironically, as the relationship develops, we become more self-conscious about how we behave in bed because we know that afterward we have to live out our daily lives with our partners, who now know more about the "real" us. We may feel that if we act too abnormally in bed, or express a desire to do something new sexually, that our partners will be upset or will view us differently.

In both cases, the end result can be the development of a sexual routine that becomes a little, well, boring. More specifically, the routine is safe. After being with someone for a while, you know what will get him off and he knows what will get you off. It's easy to resort to these techniques simply because they work. Also, by sticking to a few key activities, you don't risk raising any issues that might be a problem for either of you to address.

Sex as and when it happens

It's fine to like a few specific sexual activities. It's fine if you have a sexual schedule where you have sex on specific days or at specific times. Most of us have busy lives, and often it just happens that we fall into these kinds of patterns. But if you and your partner find yourselves just kind of going through the motions—even if they're pleasurable motions—then perhaps you might want to think about changing things a little.

How? Well, there are several ways. Try surprising your guy by initiating sex at an unexpected time. Or you might present him with a nicely wrapped gift of a new sex toy you think would be fun to try. Planning a romantic getaway can also give your sagging sex life a jolt as can simply doing something different the next time you're in bed. Try a different position. Use a new technique for getting off. Introduce fun back into your sex play.

The green-eyed monster

Many of us think that once we're in relationships all those insecurities we have when we're dating (Does he like me? Am I the only one he's sleeping with?) will magically disappear. Surprise, they don't. In fact, jealousy can be a bigger problem in relationships than it is in dating situations. Why? Because there's more at stake. If you think your partner is interested in someone else, or that someone is interested in him, you may fear your relationship is in danger.

How to cope with jealousy

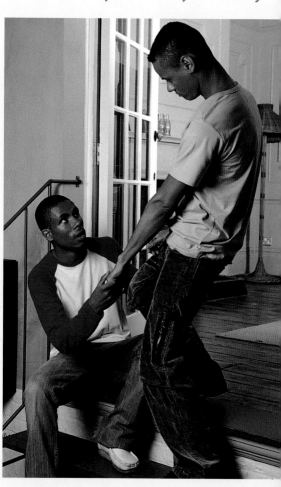

THE FIRST STEP in dealing with feelings of jealousy is telling your partner how you feel and why, even if you think he should already know.

This jealousy may even extend to his exes or his friends. You may find yourself getting anxious whenever he talks about past boyfriends, or becoming worried when he goes out with his buddies for a drink. But unless you have a real reason to think things are rocky between the two of you, your fears are almost assuredly based on your own insecurities.

If you find that jealousy is creeping into your relationship, ask yourself what you're really worried about. If you can pinpoint an actual problem, discuss it with your partner and see what can be done to correct the situation. If your fears are all about you, though, then ask yourself why you're allowing them to control your emotions, and take steps to deal with them so that they don't cause bigger problems in your relationship.

WORKING THROUGH DIFFICULT moments will ultimately make your relationship stronger because it creates feelings of trust and safety between you and your partner.

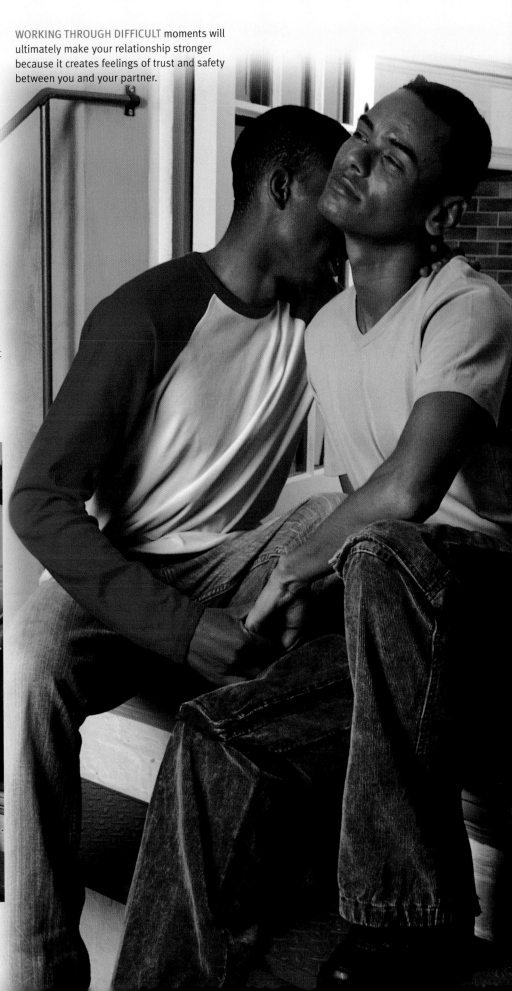

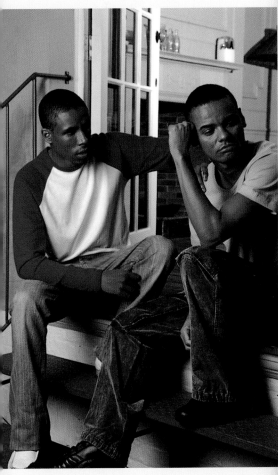

IT'S COMMON FOR a partner to react to your feelings of jealousy by being surprised or defensive. Try to listen to him without getting angry.

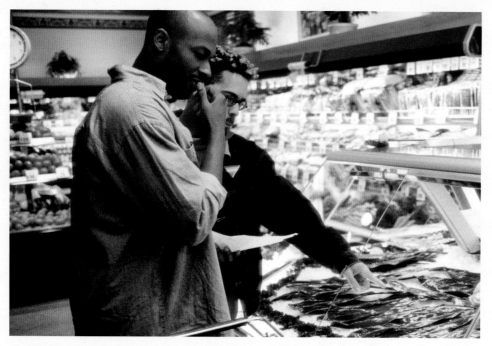

WE ALL WANT and need different things from our relationships. Define yours on what actually works for you and your partners, not on what you see other people doing or what you think you're supposed to do. The secret is to be yourselves.

relationship, there are ways to accommodate these desires. But it's important that ground rules for sexual behavior be established and that both partners follow them to avoid misunderstandings.

Three's company
Let's say that you and your partner agree that both of you are allowed to have sex with others outside the relationship. But on what conditions? Is it only when you're out of town? Are there only certain sexual acts that you or he are okay to engage in outside the relationship? Can it be only with people you don't know? Or, turning the dilemma around, only with people you do know? Are you going to tell each another about your encounters or will you have a don't ask/don't tell policy?

There are all kinds of questions you need to address when considering opening up your relationship. You also need to think about what you're going to do if one, or both of you, decides that non-monogamy is too difficult to handle. This is why being able to communicate with your partner is so important. Non-monogamy requires ongoing discussion and sometimes negotiation, and if you can't talk about what you want and how you're feeling, there's no way it's going to work for you.

Some couples address the desire for additional sexual partners, not by having sex outside the relationship, but by introducing three-ways into their relationships. This is discussed in more detail in the section on group sex (see pages 144–147).

SOME COUPLES add another person to their relationship. This introduces new issues and concerns that need to be addressed openly by everyone involved, so good communication is absolutely necessary to making these situations work.

Party time
Celebrating our relationships is important. Not only is it fun but it reinforces the bond at the heart of any partnership, and reminds us of what we get from being with someone else. Commitment ceremonies, weddings, anniversary and holiday celebrations, and even parties just to celebrate the life you share, are all ways of reaffirming relationships. Whether it's an intimate dinner for two, or a bash with everyone you know, make a point of celebrating the important events of your life as a couple.

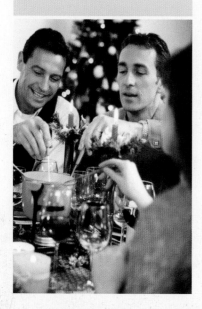

Open relationships
The traditional image of a couple is two people who are committed to each other emotionally and sexually. The concept of monogamy is often at the center of how we define a successful, healthy relationship. After all, if you're committed to someone you should want to be sexual only with that one guy, right?

For many of us this is true. A lot of couples do find that being monogamous is important to them. They find that being exclusive sexually makes the relationship stronger in other areas. Also, it prevents a lot of problems by removing feelings of insecurity and doubt. And on a purely practical level, being sexual with just one person eliminates any worries about contracting STDs and makes safer sex unnecessary (assuming both partners are free of STDs).

But some couples find that being monogamous doesn't work for them. When this happens, new rules for the relationship need to be created. If one or both partners are secretly having sex outside the relationship, then something is wrong and the reasons for the infidelity need to be addressed, and the viability of the relationship evaluated. If, however, partners recognize that one or both of them is interested in sex outside the

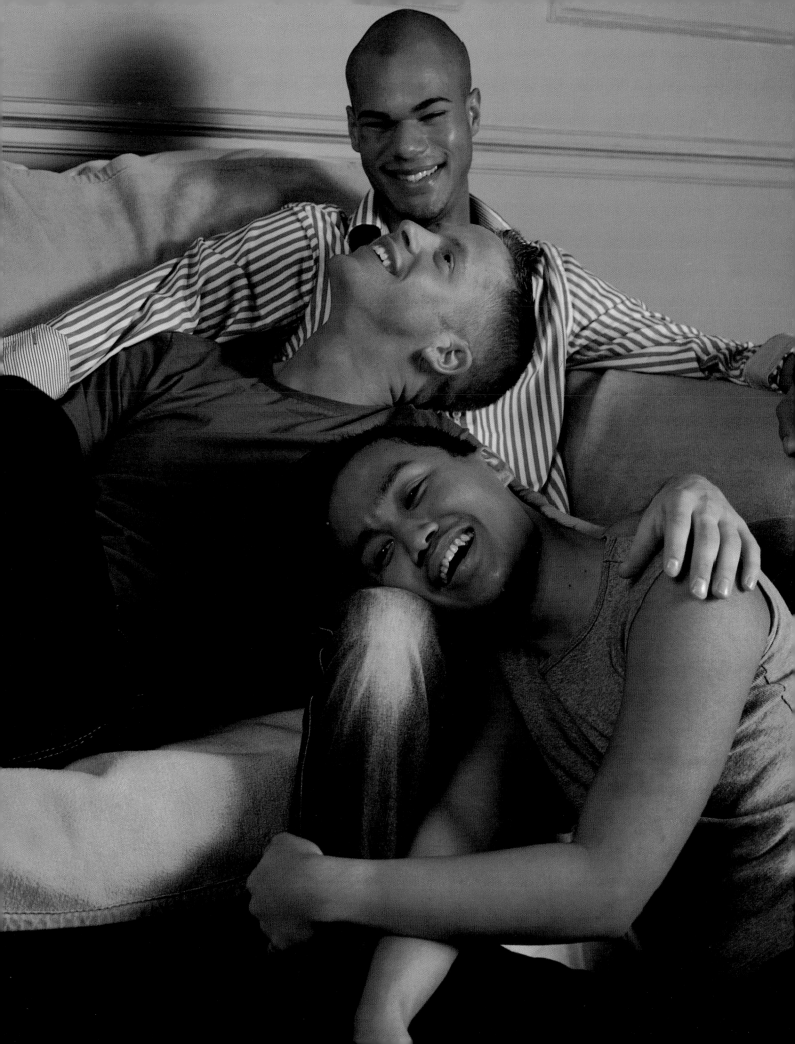

Rejection

Coping when your advances have been rebuffed

One of the biggest obstacles to romantic and sexual fulfillment is the fear of rejection. This can range from being afraid to ask someone out on a date, to avoiding truly intimate relationships with others because it means making ourselves too vulnerable. However it is manifested in our lives, the end result is that it prevents us from getting what we want. So the sooner we learn to recognize fear-based behaviors—both in ourselves and in others—and learn how to deal with them, the sooner we can get on with establishing rewarding relationships and having satisfying sexual encounters.

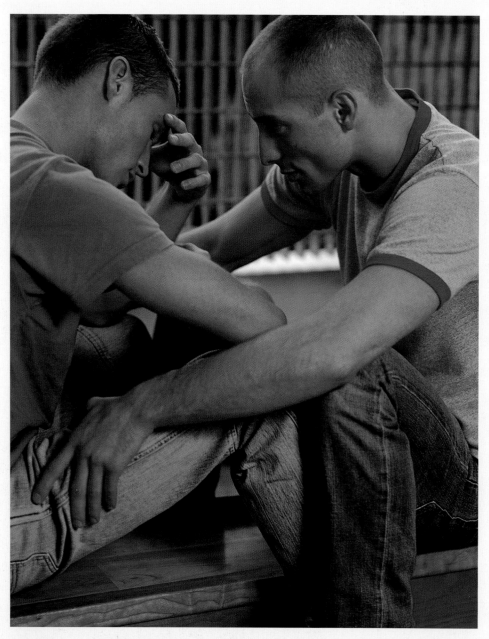

SHARING YOUR FEELINGS of rejection with a friend will reassure you that just because you've been turned down this time, doesn't mean you'll be rejected *every* time. Cheer up and get back out there.

Perceiving rejection

In its purest form, rejection is being told "no." This expression can occur in our lives in many different guises, including "No, I don't want to go out with you," "No, I don't want to continue seeing you," or perhaps "No, I'm not interested in having sex with you." Sometimes it's even more subtle: a cruise that's returned with a sneer, a promise to call that never materializes, a sexual advance rebuffed or ignored.

The rejection, though, isn't the real problem. In fact, the problem is how we perceive the rejection. Instead of hearing "No, I don't want to have dinner with you," what we really hear is "What could possibly make you think I would want to spend two hours of my time with someone like you?" And when a potential one-night stand decides to go home with someone else, we take it as absolute proof that we are, hands down, the most sexually unappealing person in the room.

No, rejection isn't fun. But most of the time the rejection is about the other person. Really, it is. We forget sometimes that just because we're attracted to someone, he isn't necessarily going to be attracted to us. The point is, rejection is almost always someone saying "I'm really sorry, but for reasons having nothing to do with who you are as a person I don't find you romantically or sexually enticing." (Unfortunately, in real life they usually don't put it this gently.)

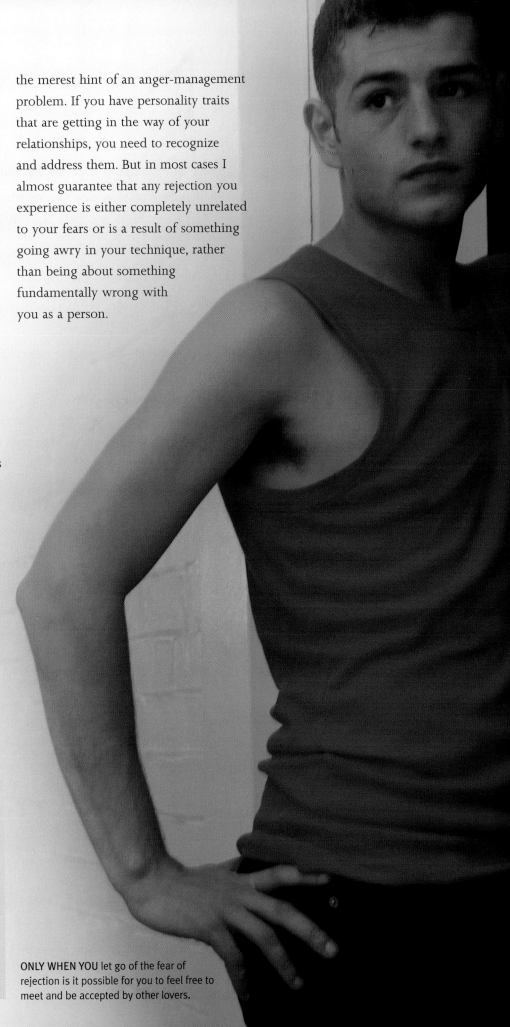

Confronting rejection head-on

Being turned down or breaking up is the disappointing result of two people not being on the same wavelength. Most of us, though, turn it into an opportunity to compose a laundry list of everything we don't like about ourselves: our extra 20 pounds, our regrettable fashion sense, our tendency toward shyness. Whatever it is we personally fear might make us romantic and sexual duds becomes magnified a million times when we find ourselves being rejected. "See," we tell ourselves, "my penis really isn't big enough." "My ex was right," we think. "I really don't know how to tell a joke."

In reality, the guy who turned you down probably has a totally unrelated reason for doing so. You're taller than he is. Maybe you look like the first guy who broke his heart. Perhaps he only dates Asians/twinkies/bears/guys with bald spots. What I'm trying to say is this: Getting rejected happens to everyone one time or another, and understanding that it has very little to do with anything truly important is crucial to being able to handle it and move on.

Now, if you find yourself being turned down or dumped repeatedly, you may have to take a closer look at yourself. There certainly are some things that might make you less appealing to other men—perhaps a nasty habit of getting falling-down drunk, a negative attitude about everything, or maybe the merest hint of an anger-management problem. If you have personality traits that are getting in the way of your relationships, you need to recognize and address them. But in most cases I almost guarantee that any rejection you experience is either completely unrelated to your fears or is a result of something going awry in your technique, rather than being about something fundamentally wrong with you as a person.

Fear of failing

Even more potentially damaging than outright rejection is letting our lives be controlled by a fear of it happening. Too many men don't put themselves out there or don't go for what they really want because they're overwhelmed by the fear that they'll fail. The next time you're considering asking someone out and you find yourself in the "What if he says no?" frame of mind, try instead to think about "What if he says yes?" Imagine what could happen if he does—the fantastic sex, the Sunday mornings in bed, the great conversation over dinner. Maybe he'll still say no, but at least when you approach him you'll do so with a positive attitude, and that can make all the difference.

ONLY WHEN YOU let go of the fear of rejection is it possible for you to feel free to meet and be accepted by other lovers.

Relationship break-ups

Why breaking up is hard to do

Whether you've been dating for a few weeks or living together for many years, the end of a relationship is seldom easy. Coming to the realization that you and a partner aren't meant to be together often involves making some hard decisions, facing some disappointment, and going through a period of sadness and adjustment. Sudden and unexpected break-ups can be particularly difficult, but even if you've seen it coming for some time, losing a partner brings up emotions and reactions that need to be addressed before you can move on with your life.

What went wrong?

Most of us have been involved in break-ups at some point and it's safe to say they aren't moments we look back on fondly. Even when the decision to end a relationship is mutual, you're usually left feeling pretty bad about things. And if you're the one who gets dumped you might feel especially awful, particularly if the break-up comes out of the blue.

When a dating relationship ends it's usually because you've spent enough time together for one or both of you to realize that things aren't going to progress any further. Perhaps the sexual chemistry just isn't there, or maybe you find you have different goals or different perspectives on important issues. Whatever the reason, when it's time to end a dating relationship the best thing to do is part ways, and take stock of what you've learned from the experience about yourself, and about what you want and don't want in a partner.

Time to split up?

It isn't always obvious that it's time to end a relationship. Sometimes our attitudes toward our partners and to our relationships are affected by unrelated things, such as depression, stress at work, dissatisfaction with other areas of our lives, and even health concerns. Instead of dealing with these problems, we blame our partner for things going wrong, and decide to end the relationship, when actually spending a little more time pinpointing the real cause of our unhappiness would have revealed the root of the problem. So before you decide to break up with a partner ask yourself why you're thinking of doing it. If all you can come up with is a list of superficial reasons, it might be that you need to reexamine your motives.

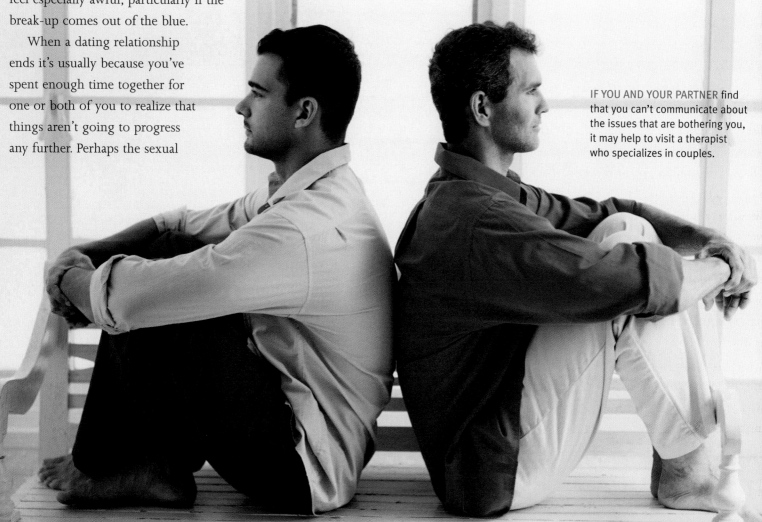

IF YOU AND YOUR PARTNER find that you can't communicate about the issues that are bothering you, it may help to visit a therapist who specializes in couples.

Break-ups involving long-term relationships are, of course, more difficult. Unless there's a sudden event that causes the break-up (such as an affair), the end of a long relationship is usually a gradual thing. It's not unusual for relationships to unravel slowly, often with neither partner being overtly aware that it's happening. There may be general feelings of dissatisfaction or unease for quite some time before the realization that things just aren't working anymore arrives.

New beginnings

Here's the single most important thing I can tell you about break-ups, no matter how long the relationship: The end of a relationship doesn't mean that the experience was a waste of time. Too often we use the word "failure" in discussing or thinking about break-ups. Break-ups are not the result of a failure; they are the result of a realization that the relationship either was simply not working in the first place, or is no longer working because of a change in circumstances. No relationship is a waste of your time—as long as you learn something from it.

The biggest mistake men make when dealing with a break-up is obsessing over the why. Why did this happen? Why did he leave? Why couldn't we make it work? Yes, you should examine why a break-up occurred. What you shouldn't do is pick it apart endlessly. Don't relive every disagreement, and every time when things weren't perfect, looking for The Problem. Chances are, the reason for the break-up is apparent. If it isn't, try to discuss it with your ex. If he won't, or if he gives you vague answers, then it may very well be about some issue of his. Let it go as much as you can. But don't blame yourself.

If you're the one to initiate a break-up, it's important to be honest with your partner about why. If this is someone you've dated for three months and you're dumping him because he listens to awful music, is wretched in bed, and doesn't clip his toenails, you might want to be diplomatic and say something general. You don't

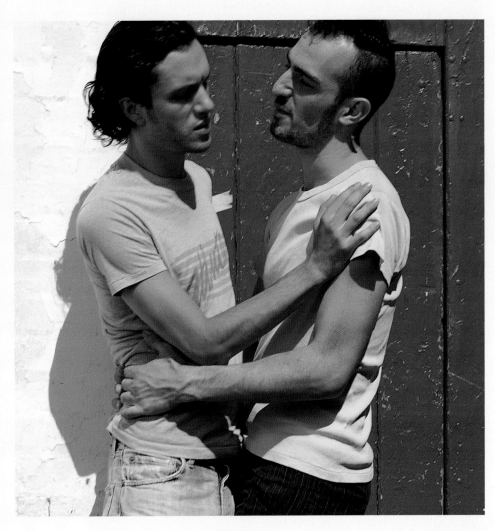

need to be cruel. But if this is someone you've been with for a while and have shared a lot with, you do owe it to him to tell the truth, even if it's difficult for you to say and for him to hear.

Time for change

In examining the break-up of a long-term relationship, the question is often "how could something that was going so well turn into something that wasn't working?" The answer to that is, people change. We should all be changing as we learn more about ourselves and explore our interests. One of the best things about relationships is watching a partner become more and more the person he's supposed to be. But sometimes two people change in incompatible ways, and when that happens a relationship that might have worked a year, three years, or even many years earlier, doesn't work anymore.

THINGS CAN START to go wrong when the two people in a partnership find they're no longer relating to each other in the way they were at the start.

The blame game

It's very tempting to want to blame someone when a relationship ends, particularly if you're the one who was dumped. Having someone to point a finger at makes the feelings of anger, disappointment, and possibly even embarrassment easier to handle. But not for long. Being mad at someone is ultimately just as self-destructive as the feelings we're trying to cover up. A better option is to indulge yourself in your feelings for a specific period of time—a weekend, or a week if you're really mad. After that, have a cleansing ritual (burning his photograph is good) and let it go.

It's not the end of the world

Usually the hardest part of a break-up is not the break-up itself but life after it. That first night when you go to bed alone, or the first morning when you wake up and realize you don't have him to talk to, can be devastating. Your life has changed and with it the routine that you maybe have had for a long time.

It's important to give yourself time to mourn the loss of a relationship. This doesn't mean feeling depressed and dwelling on the break-up; it means allowing yourself to be sad about the loss you've experienced. Even if a relationship you've shared was a bad one, a break-up is still a loss. And if your relationship was one in which you sacrificed who you were for the sake of the other person, you might find yourself angry and sad over the time you gave up for him. This is okay. In fact, it's very healthy.

Making the break

No one wants to hurt someone's feelings, but it's important not to stay in a relationship just because that seems easier than going through a break-up. If you're telling yourself that you'll end things when the holidays are over, when he's less depressed, or when you have enough money to move out, it's time to stop stalling. Don't let excuses stand between you and doing something you know you need to do. Sit your partner down and tell him how you feel. It's going to be difficult whenever you do it, and putting it off is just being afraid of facing the changes a break-up will bring. If you need to, set up a network of friends to help you through, whether by loaning you money, giving you a place to stay, or just being moral support.

You may find it easier to make the break if you know that after a certain period of down time without any contact, you can plan to meet on neutral ground to say anything you might want to say. Giving each other time before doing this allows you to process your feelings, and makes it easier to stay non-confrontational. It's okay to be sad, but don't start rehashing what happened or accusing each other of anything. This is your first step to forming a friendship beyond your old relationship, so acknowledge that things are different now. Focus on what you enjoy about each other and see if you can move forward.

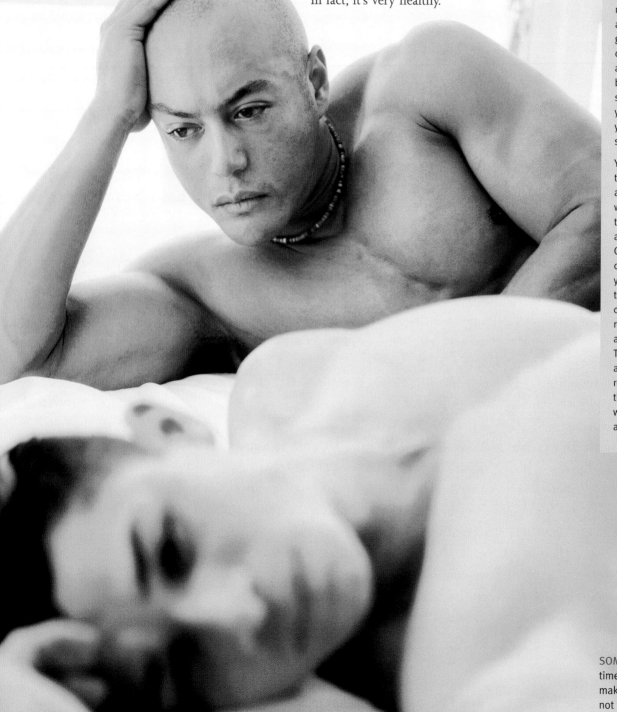

SOMETIMES IT CAN be helpful to have time apart from your partner while you make a decision about whether or not to end a relationship.

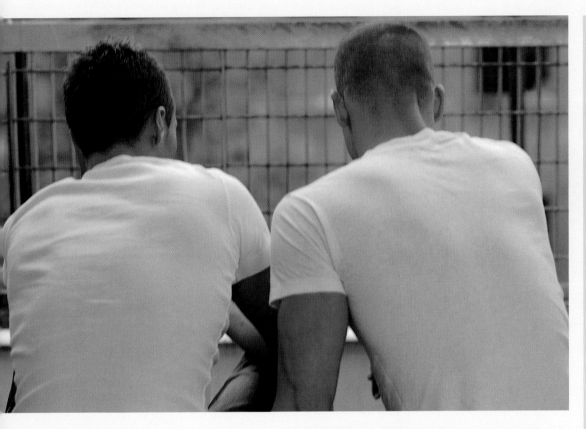

A clean slate

One thing that can help in starting life after a break-up is not dating. Often the temptation is to throw yourself back into the dating scene immediately, as a way of "getting over" your ex. Really all you're doing is looking for validation that you're still attractive to other men, but this is not particularly useful. You need some time to let go of the past relationship and to regroup.

There are no rules about how much time you take before dating again. Only you will know when it's time. But, just as some men start dating too soon, others put it off too long. They may convince themselves that it's because they will never find something as good as what they had or they say they're happy being single. That's okay, but it's important to know when you're using excuses to avoid confronting your fears.

What you had with one man is not what you will have with another. If you had a great relationship, don't think that you can never have another one. And if your previous relationship was a nightmare, don't assume that your next one will be. But in both cases having subsequent

WE ALL LEARN a lot from relationships and, by turning an unpleasant experience into one that teaches you something about yourself, you will take away as much from the experience as possible.

rewarding partnerships will require that you leave some aspects of your previous relationships behind and move forward with a positive outlook. Hanging on to them, even if they were good, succeeds only in creating insurmountable obstacles to achieving happiness.

The ex-factor

Some of us are able to maintain friendships with our past lovers; others would just as soon drink boiling oil as stay in contact. It's not uncommon for gay men to have in their circle of friends guys they dated or had long-term relationships with. Whatever happens, it's important to have a no-contact period with your ex. It sounds harsh, but talking to each other, even when you're concerned about each other, makes it very difficult to sever the emotional ties that need to be cut. You can still like your ex. You can still care for him and want him to be happy. But when you first split, you both need time alone.

Moving on

Looking ahead to a life without your partner can sometimes seem like a daunting and impossible task. But moving on is important and there are some things that you can do to make the transition easier for yourself.

• Spend time with friends. Yes, it's a distraction of sorts but more importantly it will remind you that there are people in your life who care about you.

• Focus on you. Treat yourself to new clothes or a vacation. Sign up for a class you've always wanted to take. Spend a day at a spa having everything done.

• Get out of the house. Most of us tend to become hermits after we break up with someone. Don't sit at home feeling bad. Get out there and enjoy life.

• Don't call him. You need time apart with no contact. If you find yourself tempted to call, call a friend instead.

• Clean the house. Put reminders of him away. Maybe later on you can put the photographs back up, but for now they need to be out of your sight.

• Stay away from the alcohol. Drinking will just make you dwell on what's happened and make you feel worse, so lay off the sauce for a little while.

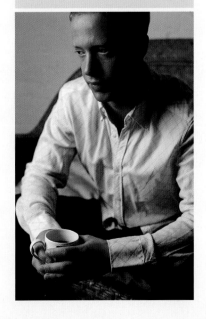

Beating depression

Fighting back for yourself

Not surprisingly, sexual happiness and fulfillment is directly related to your overall mental state. The more positive your general outlook is the more likely you are to find yourself in healthy relationships and to have enjoyable sexual encounters. Conversely, if your overall mood is negative, the more likely you are to become involved in negative situations and to engage in potentially risky sexual behavior. By understanding what depression is, how it develops, and how it can be dealt with, we take responsibility for our emotional well-being and the health of our sexual lives.

All in the mind?

If you find yourself in a negative situation, removing yourself from it can be a difficult task. Monitoring your overall emotional health can provide a helpful indication of how you feel about your sex life, and understanding your moods can help you comprehend how and why you behave the way you do in sexual situations.

To do so, you must use your brain. The brain is a remarkable thing. It acts as the processing center for our thoughts and experiences, turning out moments of pleasure, grief, happiness, and every other emotion human beings are capable of having. When it comes to sex, the brain is responsible for taking all the various tastes, smells, sounds, sights, and sensations we experience and turning them into pleasure and arousal. More than our genitals, the brain is our primary sexual organ, although few of us think about it that way when we're lost in lovemaking.

The same organ that can create such intense pleasure can also produce moments of darkness. Just as certain stimuli can result in feelings of joy and happiness, others can end in fear, anxiety, sadness, and intense feelings of despair. When these feelings persist, we become depressed.

Get the balance right

Depression has many causes, many of which are a result of chemical imbalances in the brain, due either to natural causes or to interruptions in brain function caused by outside influences, such as drugs and alcohol. However it is caused, depression can have devastating effects, rendering a person incapable of seeing life in a positive way, making him feel completely overwhelmed by unhappiness or simply exhausted by trying to fight the depression.

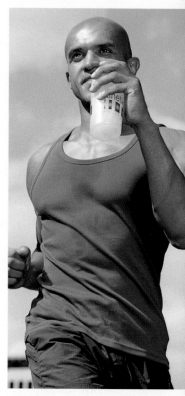

AS WELL AS keeping you fit, regular physical activity helps combat stress and depression.

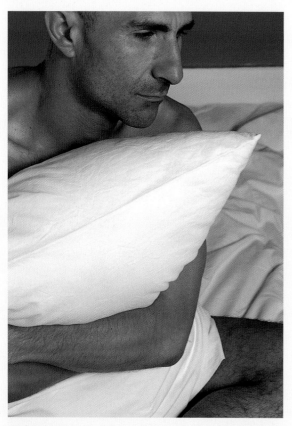

IT IS IMPORTANT to recognize when depression is limiting your capacity for happiness and satisfaction in your sexual and romantic lives.

Leave me alone!

Recognizing signs of depression isn't always easy. Some common symptoms of depression are really just magnified versions of ordinary, everyday emotions. But in general, the following are the warning signs of depression, so be sure to look out for them:

• Decreased interest in spending time with friends or in doing activities you used to enjoy.

• An often overwhelming feeling that nothing is really worth doing.

• Increased use of alcohol and/ or drugs or even an increase in food consumption, particularly of sugars and carbohydrates, to create changes in mood.

• Increased need for sleep, which isn't due to other identifiable physical causes.

• An inability to begin new projects or finish existing projects due to a lack of interest.

Many gay men find themselves battling against depression for various reasons, including issues related to homophobia, coming out, and living in situations where they feel their gayness is not accepted. Frustration over relationships, and in particular feeling incapable of finding them, is often associated with depression in gay people.

Addressing issues head-on

You may conclude that you are depressed because you can't find a partner or because things aren't going well in an existing relationship. While this may be true, it's also possible that you can't find a partner or are having trouble in a relationship because you're depressed.

Whatever the case, the underlying depression needs to be addressed before you can see what you need to do next. This means understanding that depression has physical origins and can be addressed in various ways, ranging from therapy to medication. Unfortunately, many people (and non-gay people are just as susceptible to depression as gay people) still see depression as something they should just be able to "get over" through sheer willpower or, worse, something they should be ashamed of and hide.

Nothing could be further from the truth. Yes, we all experience brief periods where we just want to be left alone, feel sad, and eat pint after pint of ice cream. Usually these spells last no more than a couple of days. But when you find yourself almost constantly overwhelmed by the feeling that nothing matters and nothing is going to change, there's something deeper going on. Then it's time to speak to a mental-health professional and find out what's happening.

Depression and sex

When it comes to sex, being depressed can have two opposing effects. It can make you shut down sexually to the point where you might not even want to think about sex. But it can also create the need to have as much sex as possible, because sex releases chemicals that create feelings of well-being. Although short-lived, these can offset the negative effects of depression. Unfortunately, as depression worsens, the need for sexual stimulation can become more frequent, resulting in sexual addiction or compulsion. Then sex becomes something to cover up your real feelings, robbing it of any true emotional satisfaction.

You gotta have good friends

Okay, so you're depressed. What are you going to do about it, sit around and stuff your face with pound cake? Put on all your moodiest albums and boo hoo? No, at least not for more than a day or two.

• TAKE THE DOG FOR A WALK
Staying inside when you feel depressed is the worst thing you can do. You need to get your body moving and remove yourself from an unhappy atmosphere. So take Spot for a run in the park. Go to the gym. Walk on the beach. Get out into the world.

• PICK UP THE PHONE, PART 1
Misery loves company, right? So make some calls. Talk to your friends. And I mean your real friends, the ones who will let you sob for a while and then come over, make you shower and get dressed, and take you out dancing. Make sure you have a support network for when you need it.

• CLEAN YOUR HOUSE
When you feel miserable, you tend to let things go. So pull out the vacuum cleaner. Get rid of dirty dishes. Make your surroundings reflect how you want to feel.

• DON'T SELF-MEDICATE
Half a box of chocolate chip cookies is okay, but lay off alcohol and drugs. Depressants like alcohol and pot will make you even more weepy, while stimulants such as coke and Ecstasy will make you forget your troubles for a while but bring them crashing down even harder when the high wears off.

• PICK UP THE PHONE, PART 2
Know when your depression is more than just a bad mood. If you feel like you just can't handle it any more, it's time to get help. Call your local health center, look in the local queer paper, or ask your friends who they see.

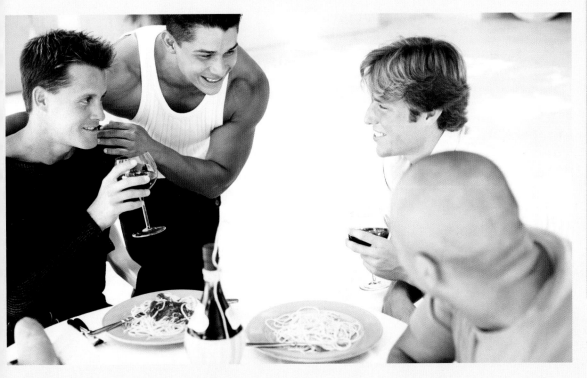

SPENDING TIME WITH friends doing the things you enjoy can help maintain a positive outlook on life.

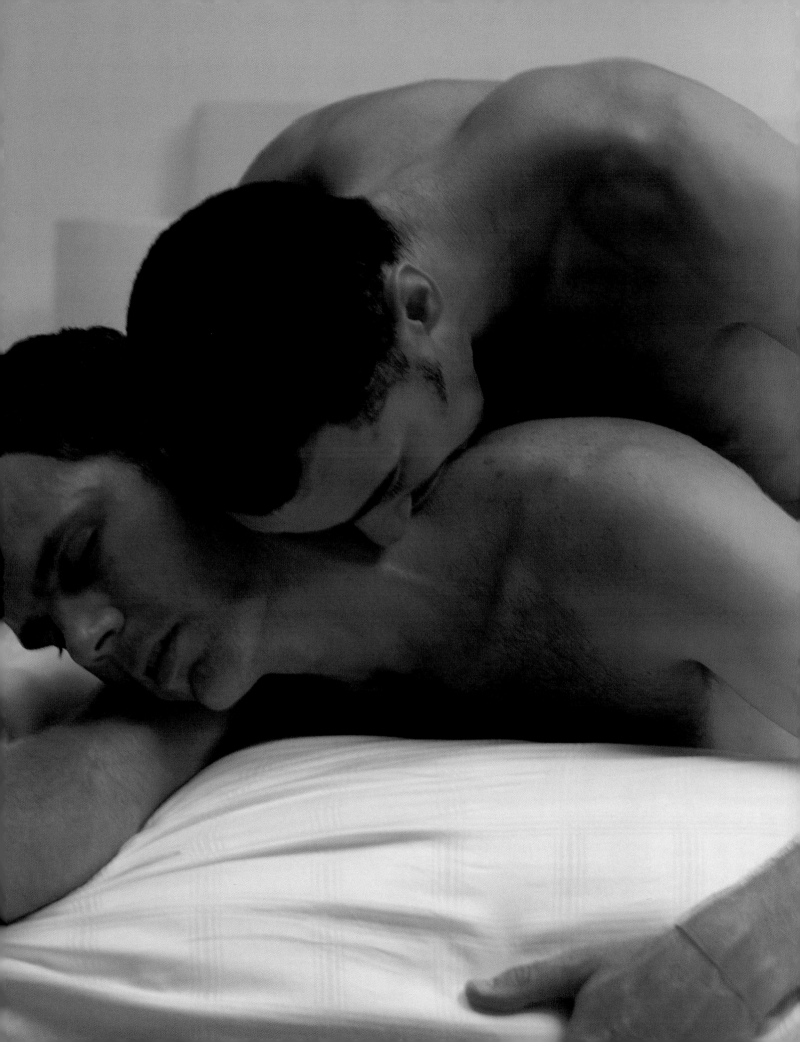

4 Sex: doing it

Great lovers aren't born; they're made. Becoming
a great lover takes practice, passion, and, most
importantly, an understanding of what brings pleasure
to you and to your partners. Learning how to get
the most out of your sexual encounters is something
anyone can master. All it takes is a willingness to
be open to the possibilities within yourself.

Safer sex

Getting the message across

In 1992, I wrote one of the first books about the AIDS crisis for young people. At the time, the rate of HIV infection among people under the age of 25 was growing at an alarming rate. Nearly a decade later it had declined significantly, to the point where it seemed that maybe the message of safer sex had gotten through. But in the last two or three years, the trend has reversed. Suddenly incidents of new infection in young people, particularly in young gay men, have increased even more quickly than they did the first time around. Apparently, the message needs to be repeated.

A misnomer of sorts

Sex was never completely safe. There have always been sexually transmitted diseases such as hepatitis, herpes, gonorrhea, syphilis, and even plain old urinary tract infections and genital warts. But it's become even less "safe" since we first learned of the existence of HIV over 20 years ago. Now when we talk about safer sex we think primarily of preventing infection with the AIDS virus. We even changed the name somewhere along the line, going from "safe" to the less sure "safer." Of course, this is more accurate. Even the techniques we associate with safer sex—wearing condoms, avoiding coming into contact with body fluids,

Can I say no?

Knowing what *could* happen if you engage in a sex act does not prevent it from happening. What it does is give you facts on which to base your personal level of acceptable risk.

• The biggest barrier to practicing safer sex is being afraid to insist on it. Often, we're afraid that if we ask a guy to wear a rubber, or if we refuse to participate in potentially risky behavior, he'll lose interest or we'll spoil the mood. But is one hot sexual experience worth living the rest of your life with an STD? No, it isn't.

• Too often "mistakes" are made when we decide that some guy is so hot, or the sex we're having is so great, that we don't want to "ruin" things by saying no. Just remember that *you* are the most important person in the equation.

• You can't live your life in fear of what might happen, but you *can* learn how to minimize the risk of exposing yourself to potential STDs— as well as what to do if you become infected with one.

PLAYING AROUND WITH condoms can be a fun element of foreplay. The correct use of condoms is based on a clear understanding of the risks involved in sexual activity and how best to minimize them.

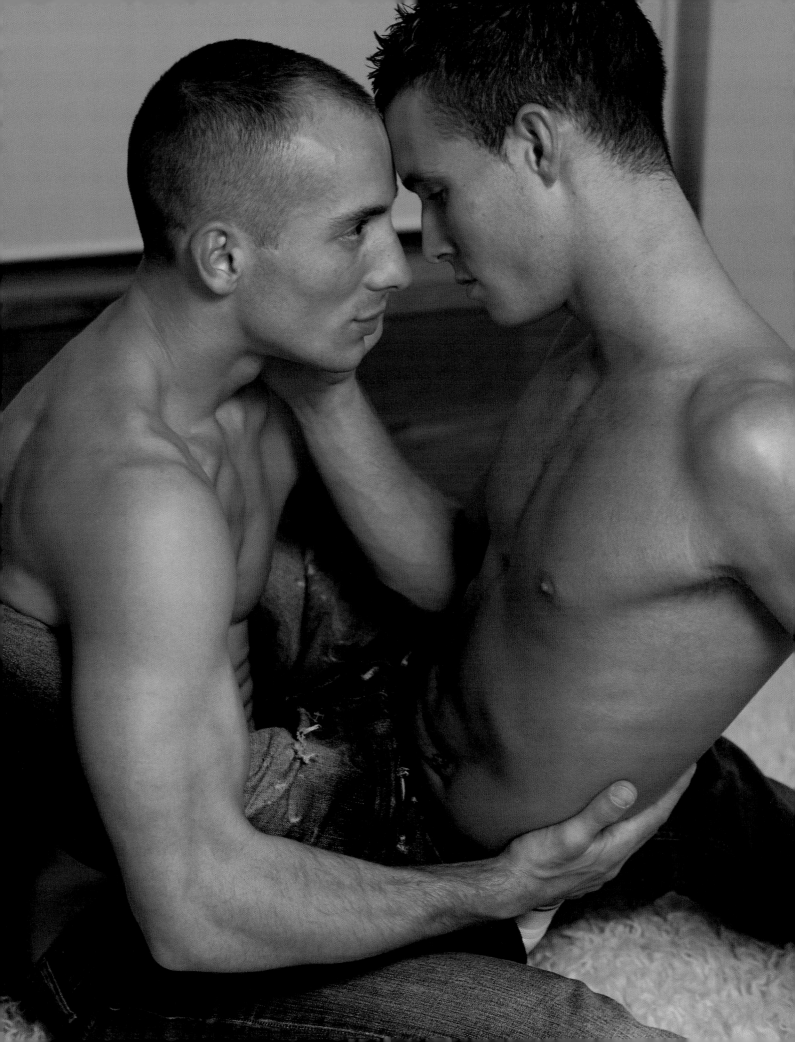

understanding the hows and the whys of transmission—can't protect us fully. Condoms break. We let our guard down. We trust someone we shouldn't have trusted. These things happen.

So then, what is "safer" sex? It's educated sex. It's understanding what engaging in sexual activity potentially exposes you to, and it's making educated choices about your health.

Understanding the basics

The basics are easy enough to understand. When you engage in sexual activity where someone else's penis is in your mouth or ass, your penis is in his mouth or ass, or either of your tongues is in the other's ass, there is the potential for transmitting viruses. Even kissing can result in the transmission of certain viruses, as can fingering someone's butt, if you then put your fingers in your mouth. Essentially, for you to become infected with HIV, the virus has to come into contact with your bloodstream and this can occur sexually if an infected guy's semen gains access to your bloodstream through cuts or scrapes in your rectum, mouth, or urethra. This makes it sound as if every time you get into bed with someone you're putting your health at risk.

In some ways you are. But that doesn't mean you shouldn't have sex, or that you can't minimize the risks. Just use your head and enjoy yourself.

What makes sex "safer"?

Obviously, the only completely safe sex is sex with yourself. But in all likelihood you will want to do it with someone else at some point. In that case, use what you know about how HIV and other viruses are spread. What would prevent their transmission?

Latex condoms, when used properly, provide the most effective barrier against sexually transmitted diseases, particularly in regard to anal sex, by containing ejaculate inside the condom. Not allowing a partner to ejaculate in your mouth minimizes (but does not completely eliminate) the potential for infection through cuts on your tongue, gums, or inside your mouth. Washing the fingers or penis after unprotected anal contact, and before subsequent oral activities, reduces the risk of transmitting viruses.

In short, use your head. There's no one thing that will make sex totally safe, but if you follow these guidelines, the likelihood of contracting a sexually transmitted disease will be greatly reduced.

Levels of risk

• Unprotected anal intercourse can expose you to infection (particularly to HIV) whether you're the active (top) or receptive (bottom) partner.

• Unprotected oral sex is less risky, but still has the potential for the transmission of not only HIV, but also gonorrhea and other STDs. There are no documented cases of HIV infection from receiving oral sex, but if the person performing oral sex has any infections in his throat, they could be passed on to you.

• Mouth-to-anus sex (rimming) is considered a minimal risk activity for transmission of HIV. However, this is an excellent way to pick up other nasties, including amoebas, giardia, hepatitis A, and perhaps even syphilis or gonorrhea.

• Masturbation with a partner is a great alternative to penetrative sex. Although there is a remote possibility of infection, should a partner's body fluids come into contact with cuts on your hands or skin, masturbating together is a relatively risk-free option.

Condom sense

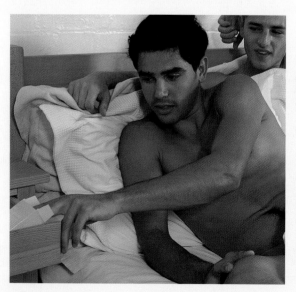

NOT ALL RUBBERS are created equal—latex condoms are the safest. "Natural" or lambskin condoms are made from a membrane that allows viruses, including HIV, to pass through.

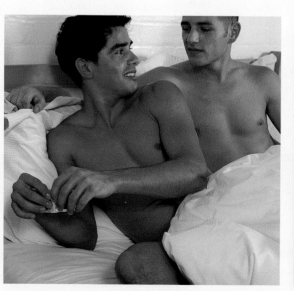

MANY PEOPLE BELIEVE that the spermicide nonoxynol-9, added to some condoms to help prevent pregnancy, will help in preventing HIV infection. It doesn't.

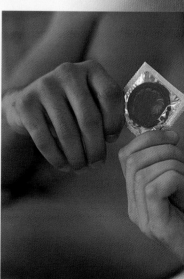

NEVER USE AN expired condom. And don't double up—two condoms seem like extra protection, but they often tear.

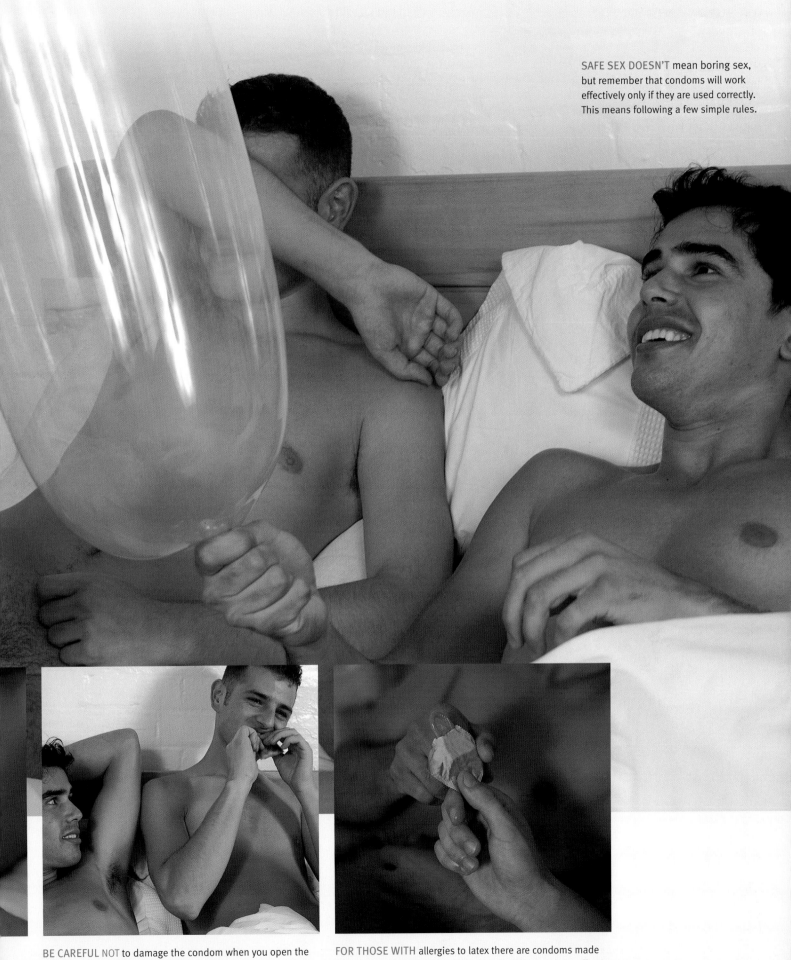

SAFE SEX DOESN'T mean boring sex, but remember that condoms will work effectively only if they are used correctly. This means following a few simple rules.

BE CAREFUL NOT to damage the condom when you open the packet. Use only water-based lubricants, because oil-based ones break down latex and can cause the condoms to fail.

FOR THOSE WITH allergies to latex there are condoms made from polyurethane, although the jury is still out on how effective these condoms are in preventing sexually transmitted diseases.

Kissing

How to kiss

Depending on who's doing it and how it's done, a kiss can be much more than just a kiss. Think about kissing your Aunt Sylvia. Now imagine kissing your favorite male actor. See the difference? It only takes a changing breath here, and a lingering there, to turn a kiss from a happy greeting into a precursor to hot, sweaty sex. So it's crucial to understand what happens when we kiss, and how to make a kiss mean what we want it to mean.

KISSING IS ONE of the most passionate and intimate acts we can share with a lover. Try little bites on his lower lip, caress his tongue with your tongue, run your fingers through his hair—let your desire be your guide.

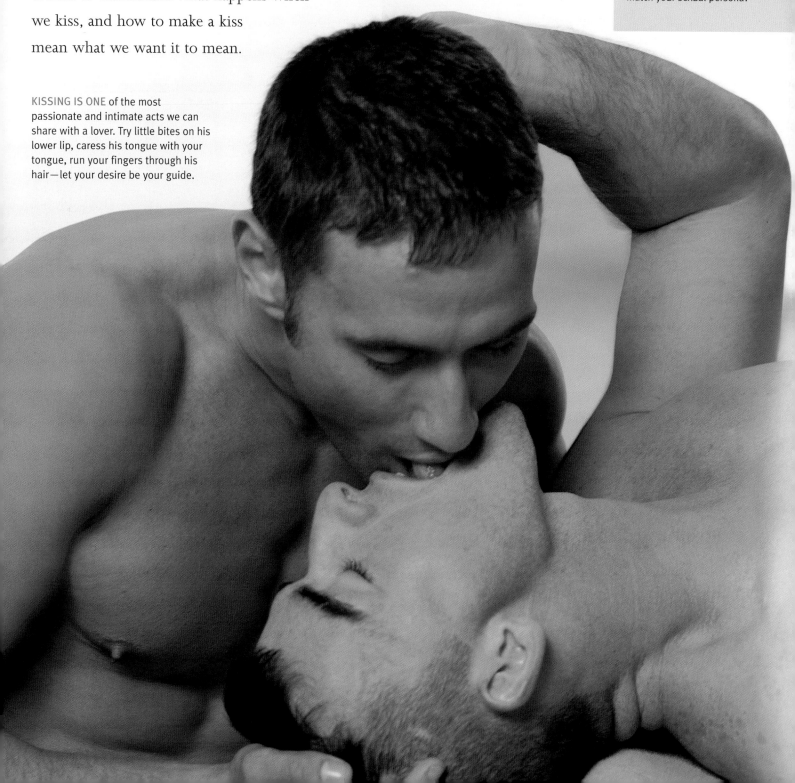

Giving and receiving

Think of a kiss as a match that starts a fire. When we kiss, we awaken our sexual response cycle. Each subsequent kiss adds fuel to this fire, causing us to grow more and more excited. As the kissing becomes more passionate, so do we. But why? What's so exciting about kissing?

You can think of kissing as having sex in miniature. Our mouths are openings to our bodies, openings through which words, food, and air move. In many ways the lips and tongue resemble sexual organs; those that open to receive and those that penetrate. When we kiss, these parts join those of our partner. Tongues slipping between parted lips is a form of touch that is a foretaste of what might come next.

Kissing is an intensely intimate experience, in some ways more intimate than sex itself. Throughout history kisses have signified lust, betrayal, friendship, death, and everything in between. Is it any wonder that some men are more upset to find out a boyfriend or partner has kissed someone else than to learn that he's slept with another guy?

Kissing as foreplay

When we think about kissing we generally envision putting mouth to mouth. But kissing can and should involve the whole body. Even in a mouth-to-mouth kiss, you can use your hands and the rest of your body to stimulate your partner and enrich the experience of the kiss. Placing a hand on the back of the neck and pulling your partner into you can be both very exciting and intimate, as can wrapping your legs around your partner's waist if you're sitting and he's standing. Pressing your erect penis against your partner while kissing (either clothed or naked) is also certain to increase arousal in you both. It pays to play around a little.

Involving the whole body in kissing becomes even more important during penetrative sex, where it can be either a precursor to the main event or an accompaniment to it. While kissing

various parts of your lover's body can put him in the mood for more, it can also help slow down the action when you want to draw things out.

So what's the difference between a good kiss and a bad kiss? Your body positioning, perhaps? Whether you have your eyes open or closed? Both of you having great breath? It's all these factors and more. In part it depends on what your partner likes. Some guys prefer tender, light, kisses, while others love wet, deep kisses

Kiss and tell?

How do you tell someone he's a bad kisser? If you don't plan on seeing him again, you don't. But if he's someone you want to keep around then you need to do something. Show him by example. Kiss him the way you want to be kissed. Once he sees what makes you hot, he'll get the idea.

The art of kissing

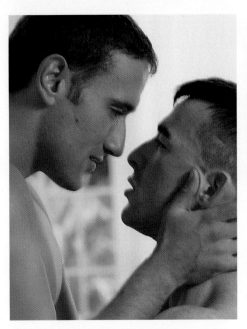

REMEMBER THE INTENSE eye contact you made when you first saw each other? Don't stop now. Gaze into your partner's eyes as you embrace.

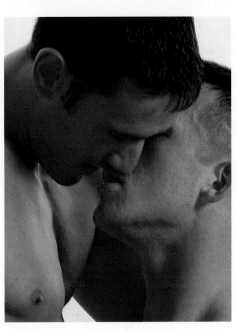

TAKE A DEEP BREATH, pucker up, and part your lips. Pull your partner toward you, grasping him seductively as your mouths meet.

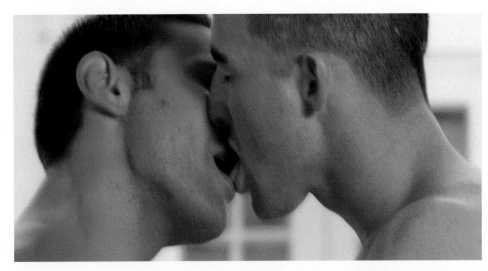

AS YOUR LIPS CONNECT, slowly slide your tongue in, tasting your partner. Keep the tempo slow, gradually increasing the pace and force. Build to a sexy crescendo that will leave him open-mouthed.

Exploratory kissing

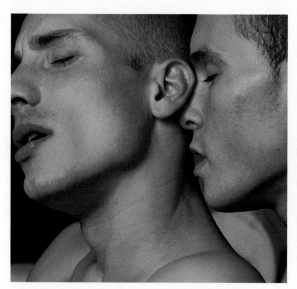

THE TOUCH OF your mouth on your partner's neck is a sensual beginning to lovemaking. Many men are aroused simply from the feel of a partner's breath on their skin.

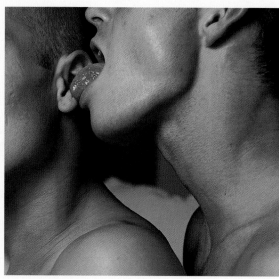

DON'T CONCENTRATE ON just one area when kissing. Use your mouth all over his body, allowing the rush of desire to flow from one place to the next.

Is good breath important?

For many men, the taste of their partner's mouth can be a real turn-on. A lot of guys, for example, love kissing someone who has just drunk whiskey or other strong-tasting drinks. Some guys enjoy the taste of cigars in a man's kiss. Very few men, though, like the taste of strong-flavored foods. If you find yourself in a kissing situation after putting away a pile of steak and onions, get yourself a shot of scotch or down a beer to help wash away any unpleasant tastes. You want your partner to be thinking of you, not your dinner.

involving lots of tongue. Many of us enjoy giving and receiving both—it just depends on how we happen to be feeling at the time.

Ultimately, a good kiss is one that achieves the kind of mood you're going for. That's why it's important to know what kind of kiss goes with which activity. It's just like picking the right wine to go with dinner. You're not going to slobber all over your lover's neck if what you're trying to do is create a mood of gentle romance. But there are other occasions when sticking your tongue down his throat and giving him a bite or two may be just what he wants. This is where instinct should kick in.

Again, it all comes down to knowing how to read your partner's moods and his desires. A good kisser knows how to use his mouth to increase a partner's arousal, sometimes teasing him and sometimes letting him know who's boss. He senses when to increase the tempo and when to linger. His kisses indicate both his own desire and his intentions, telling a partner what he's in the mood for and how he wants to do it. By learning to pick up on the signals your partner is giving out, and knowing how to respond, you'll soon be the consummate kisser.

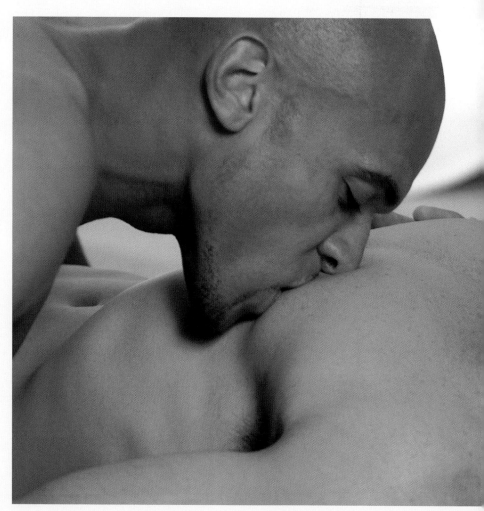

WHEN KISSING SENSITIVE areas of your partner's body—such as the nipples, genitals, or ticklish parts—create erotic tension by varying the force of your kiss. Talk to each other, so that you know exactly where to find his hot spots, sending shock waves through his body.

Mouth to mouth

Add spice to your kissing with one of these options:

• Fill your mouth with a cold drink before kissing. Allow the liquid to flow from your mouth to his.

• If your partner is lying on his back, alter the experience by kneeling beside him to kiss him.

IT ISN'T JUST your mouth that's involved in a kiss. You can use your whole body to stimulate your partner while kissing.

Massage

Releasing the pressure

Massage can certainly be erotic and even when it's not, it's an extremely intimate activity, sometimes even more intimate than sex itself. You can have sex with someone without really paying much attention to him, but it's impossible to give somebody a good massage without getting up close and personal with his body. You feel where his muscles are highly developed and where he maybe has an extra little bit of weight. You touch his scars and birthmarks and moles. You come to know every inch of him in detail, and this can be very, very pleasurable for both of you.

Setting the scene

Because massage brings you into such close contact with your partner's body, knowing how to give a good massage is important to making the experience a pleasurable one for both of you. Being able to give a good massage is a skill well worth having and, if you become good at it, your partners will be in heaven every time you touch them. Don't worry about doing it "wrong" or about not being an expert at it. All you have to do is put your hands on him and try to make him feel good. Before long you'll know just what to do.

The experience of massage begins with being comfortable. You can give a massage pretty much anywhere—on the floor, on a bed, even in the grass—as long as your partner is able to relax. So make the area where you're working pleasant. Put a soft blanket or even a fluffy sheepskin or a throw on the ground or bed. Light some candles and turn the lights down low. Burn incense. Light a fire. Play soft music. Do whatever you like to create a magical, sensuous atmosphere. What you both wear will also affect the mood. Of course, for the most sensuous experience you

Oils to spoil

Massage oils and lotions can be scented to help to create a specific mood. Lighter aromas such as lavender and vanilla promote relaxation, while mint and lemon are invigorating, and cinnamon and patchouli fuel erotic passion. You can either buy pre-made oils or make your own by adding a few drops of scent to unscented oil.

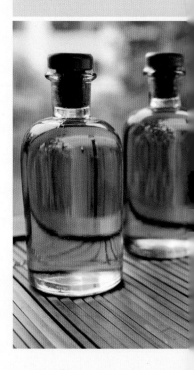

His back

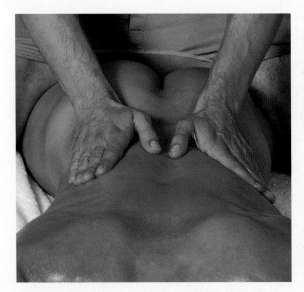

START BY PLACING your hands on either side of your partner's lower back, with thumbs aligned with his spine and the fingers spread out.

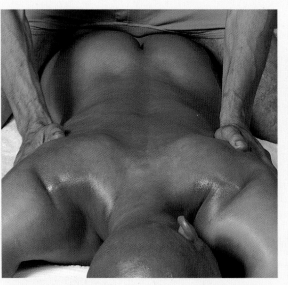

LEANING FORWARD, let your hands slide slowly up your partner's back toward his shoulders, pushing them outward before coming back down again.

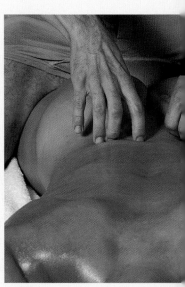

RETURN TO THE lower back and gently "comb" your partner's skin. Make little circular motions to stimulate the area.

will want to be naked, but you can also wear soft, loose clothing. The crucial thing is to be relaxed and comfortable.

Getting the right touch

Using oil or lotion makes for a much more enjoyable massage. This not only softens your skin and your partner's, it helps create smooth hand movements and adds a measure of sensuality to the experience. The smell of a luxurious oil or lotion also helps create an air of relaxation. There are many pre-made massage oils available, but you can also easily make your own. Do not use baby oil, olive oil, corn or other vegetable oils for massage, since they can leave the skin sticky and often have overwhelming scents. Also, keep in mind that some massage oils can stain clothing, so be careful to keep them away from things you don't want dirtied—or put a sheet beneath your partner to catch any stray drips.

Pain-free rubbing

Massage isn't a case of no pain, no gain. Be especially careful when working on the neck and shoulders, where exerting too much pressure or pinching can be extremely uncomfortable. Aim to *relax* your partner. Use both hands together, working the area with your fingers to ease muscle tension.

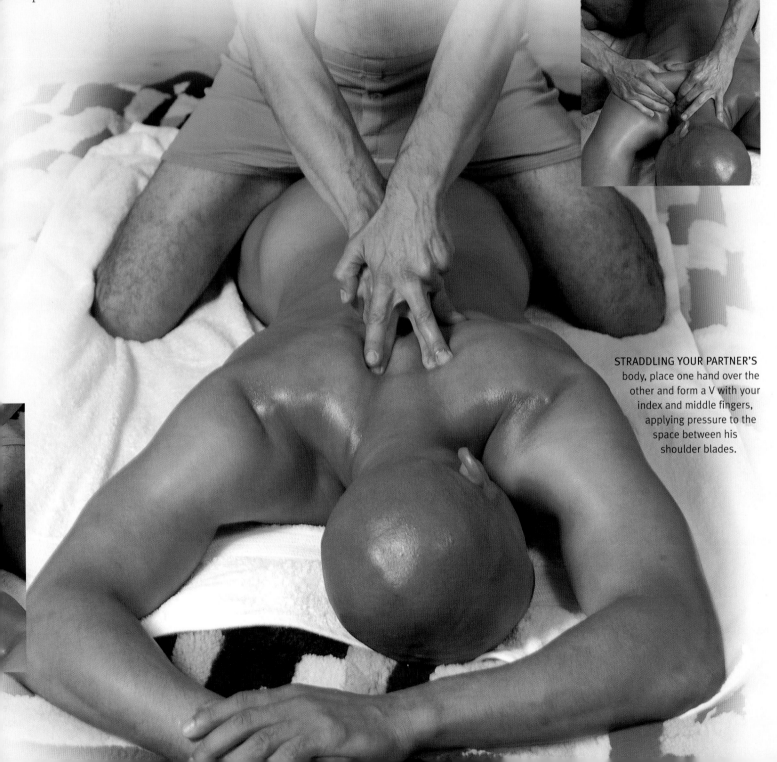

STRADDLING YOUR PARTNER'S body, place one hand over the other and form a V with your index and middle fingers, applying pressure to the space between his shoulder blades.

His shoulders

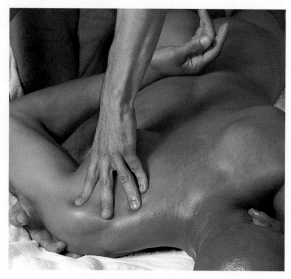

USING AN OPEN-HAND METHOD allows you to create several pressure points at once.

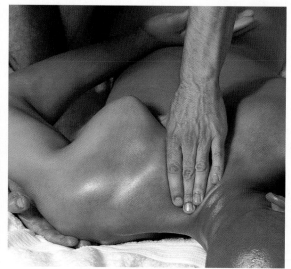

A CLOSED HAND results in a larger area of pressure on your partner's body.

Some people mistakenly believe that when it comes to massage, the old adage "the harder the better" is the secret to a sensuous rubdown. It's much more soothing and arousing if you use moderate pressure on your partner's body rather than kneading him as if you're making bread dough. Men, in particular, often go overboard when massaging, which only results in pain instead of pleasure. How do you know if you're

being too rough? Ask. And pay attention to your partner's reactions. If he keeps tensing up, chances are you need to lighten your touch a bit.

Sharing the pleasure

The massage itself can take many forms, from one that focuses on a particular body part, such as the feet or the back, to a full-body massage. The truth is, most people are happy to have any

His legs and butt

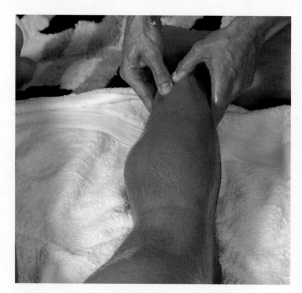

GENTLY ROTATE THE ankle, stretching the foot and massaging the hamstring area with your fingertips to relax it. Work the toes, but be careful of tickling.

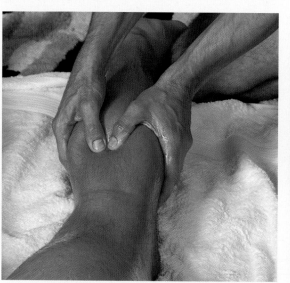

THE CALVES ARE one area where you can use greater pressure during massage. Use both hands to grasp the calf, and work the muscles with your fingers and palms.

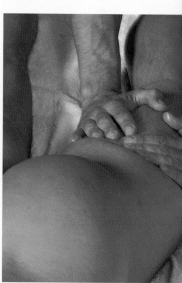

LEAN FORWARD with your hands flat as you apply pressure to the large muscles of the upper thigh.

...ind of massage at all. Having someone's hands
...n you, paying close attention to you and your
...ody, is an intensely satisfying experience.

If you decide you are going to focus on
...ne body area, really focus on it, taking time
...o bring about complete relaxation. You might
...hoose to make his shoulders the center
...f your undivided attention. Or give
...is hands or his head a slow,
...houghtful going-over. Having
...hat much time devoted to
...is body cannot fail to put
...im into a blissful state.

He'll be even more
...elighted if you decide
...o do a full-body massage.
...n this case, it's best to start
...oy positioning him on his
...stomach. Straddle his back just
...oelow his butt and start at his
...ower back, working your
...hands up along either side
...of his spine to his shoulders.
...This is usually where men have
...he most tension, so you want
...o work the area really well.

ANOTHER GOOD TECHNIQUE to use on
the thighs is paddling. Strike the area
with alternating hands, to create
a rhythmic series of movements
from the buttocks to the knee.

MASSAGING THE BUTT means getting in there and going
to work. Use a hand on each cheek and rub them in
alternating circles for the greatest effect.

YOU CAN ALSO use your fists on the buttocks, kneading
them with a rolling motion for deeper penetration. Alternate
this technique with gentle stroking.

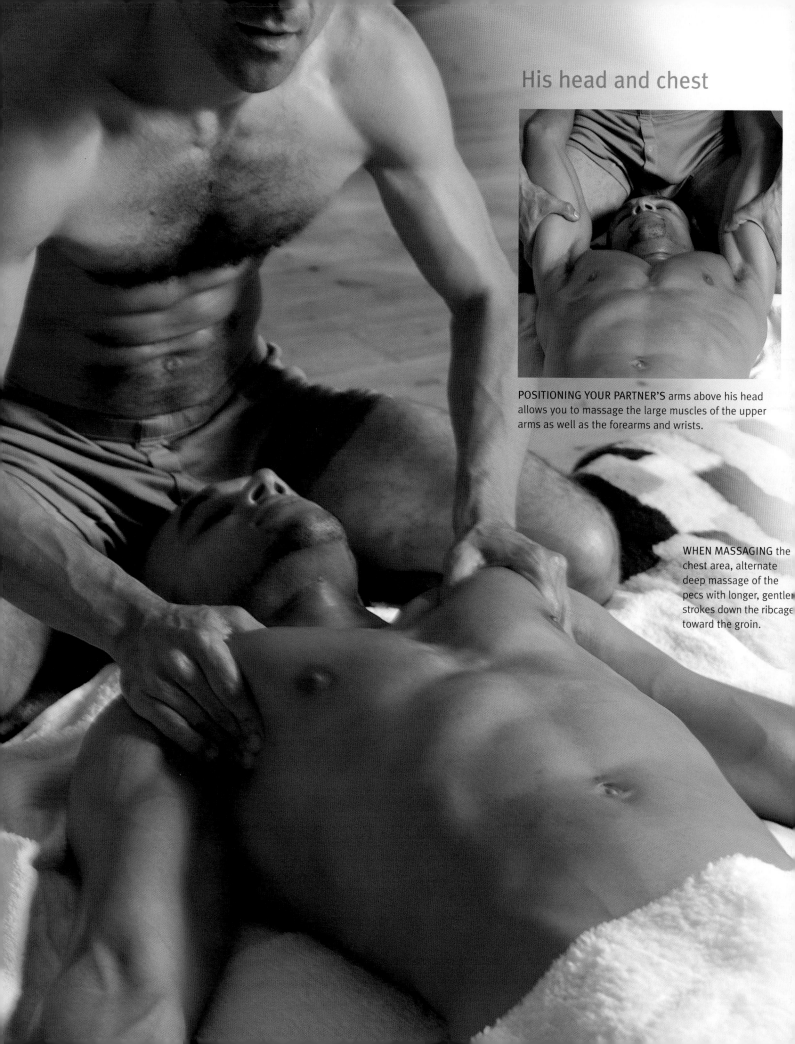

His head and chest

POSITIONING YOUR PARTNER'S arms above his head allows you to massage the large muscles of the upper arms as well as the forearms and wrists.

WHEN MASSAGING the chest area, alternate deep massage of the pecs with longer, gentler strokes down the ribcage toward the groin.

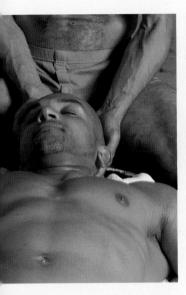

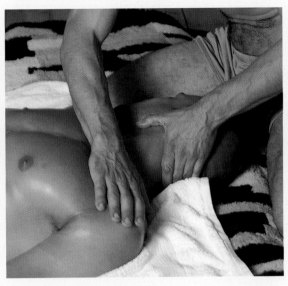

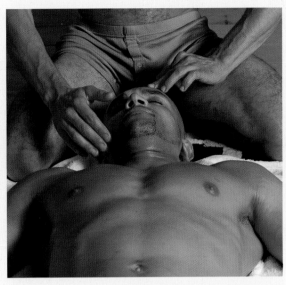

A HEAD RUB is relaxing and arousing. Cradling the head in both hands, apply direct pressure with your fingertips.

THE NECK AND shoulders should be treated as one area. Plan your strokes to move down the neck and out to the shoulders, then back again.

GENTLE TAPS OF the fingertips, accompanied by small circles and strokes across the eyelids, cheeks, and eyes, will relax his facial muscles and produce a calming effect.

Employ broad circular strokes as you move up his back, across his shoulders, and back down again. Extend the massage to his neck and head, being sure to include his scalp. As you move back down his body, let your hands move over his arms, giving them some attention as well.

At this point you might be tempted to work on his butt and make the massage a more erotic experience, but hold off for a while. You want to focus on his thighs and legs first. Massage the legs with long, firm strokes. Spend some time on his feet, rubbing them and working on his toes. You want him to relax, but you also want him to be thinking about what might be coming next.

The next stage

Now it's time to take things to the next level. Move back up to his ass. Rub the cheeks firmly. If you want to, you can throw in some kisses or little bites now. If he seems to like this, you may want to go even further, spreading the cheeks and running your fingers between them. This can, of course lead to more intimate activities like fingering or licking his anus, or possibly to anal sex, but for now let's continue with other areas of his body.

Have your partner gently roll over onto his back now. It's possible that all this massaging has gotten him aroused. If so, go for his penis and testicles, caressing him slowly. The oil on your hands and their stroking movements will create an intensely sensuous feeling, especially if you hold him tightly and slide your hand over the head of his penis and give him a gentle rub.

Or you might decide to pay some attention to his chest first. Massage it as you did his back, using firm circular motions. Let your fingertips flicker over his nipples, giving them a little pinch if you want to. Again, if he's hard and you want to take things further, now is a good time to get out of your own clothes and get into some more intimate action. Or you can keep the focus entirely on him and masturbate him or simply continue to massage him while he relaxes.

Whether your massage ends with sex or not, it's the experience of touching your partner so intimately and of giving him your undivided attention that will make this a satisfying experience for both of you. Afterward, you can prolong the pleasurable experience by relaxing and enjoying to the full the peaceful, soothing mood that you've created together.

Hand to hand

Don't let your hands neglect his hands. Interlock your fingers with his to stretch them out and loosen stiff muscles. Rotate his wrist and apply gentle pressure on his palm to remove any stiffness.

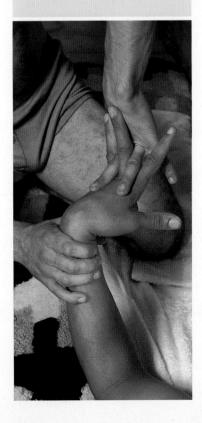

Turning him on

The things you can do to put your guy in the mood are pretty much endless, but here are a few suggestions to get you started.

• Be mysterious. Tell him to meet you at a restaurant for dinner, and then take him to a hotel for a hot night of fun.

• Be sporty. Challenge him to a wrestling match, game of pool, or card game, and make it a rule that the loser has to do what the winner wants him to do.

• Be playful. Get him to laugh by tickling him. Let it turn into some hands-on fun.

• Be seductive. Ask him to leave the room. Light a scented candle, turn on a favorite piece of music, put a heap of cushions and a bottle of wine on the floor in front of a log fire—then call him back in.

• Be sexy. Put on a strip show for him, slowly and deliberately undressing him and yourself.

• Be attentive. Treat him to a long, sensuous massage that becomes more sexual as it goes on.

• Be tender. Suggest you take a bath or shower together and give him a good, sudsy, all-over scrub.

• Be spontaneous. Surprise him by getting frisky at an unexpected time of day or in an unexpected or unusual place.

• Be bad. Show him how naughty you can be by suggesting something down and dirty.

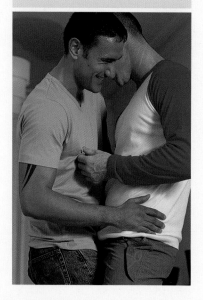

Foreplay
The prelude to lovemaking

We all know that you don't pitch in the big game until you've warmed up in the bullpen, and you don't take center stage on Broadway until you've run through a couple of renditions of Do-Re-Me. So why shouldn't you have a warm-up period when it comes to sex? You should, and that's where foreplay comes in. Before the action gets hot and heavy you need to take time to get yourself and your partner in the mood and create an atmosphere of romance. So why not try to make foreplay the main course rather than just the delicious appetizer?

Why wait?

When I was a kid I found among the books on my mother's bookshelf a battered paperback guide to sex for newlyweds. It listed a step-by-step routine that couples should follow, from undressing one another right through orgasm. There was a short section on foreplay, which basically consisted of helpful hints on breast stroking and kissing and trying not to ejaculate prematurely. It was awkward and funny, but in some ways it was also sort of right on.

Foreplay, in broad terms, is anything you do to create a sexy, romantic setting and mood that makes your interactions with your partner more enjoyable. Cynics will say it's the boring stuff you have to get through before you get to the real action, but that's an attitude held by guys trying to hide the fact that they're bad lovers.

It's true that sometimes you just want to jump right into sex. More often, though, you want a build-up. Time spent kissing your partner, touching each other, and even acting silly and laughing together all helps ease you into more intense sexual action. It creates feelings of happiness and excitement, establishes an atmosphere of both safety and freedom to explore. And ultimately, it makes sex better because it prolongs the sexual response cycle.

Foreplay can begin long before you reach the bedroom. It can start at dinner, when you hold your partner's hand or share food with him. It can begin at the movies, when you lean over and whisper in his ear, telling him how you're going to rip his clothes off when you get back to your place. Anything you say or do to get things started sexually is foreplay, because it gets you and your partner thinking about sex, and when you think, you arouse yourself emotionally.

You big tease

Remember, the whole point of foreplay is to give little hints of what's to come. In some ways it's teasing. You want your partner to know that you have big plans in store for him, but you don't want to reveal too much too quickly. It's like one of those old-fashioned strip shows where first you see a bit of leg, then maybe a bare butt. You know the whole thing is waiting behind the feathers or the fan, and you can imagine it in your mind. But not seeing it all at once makes the anticipation almost unbearable, and terribly arousing, because you can fantasize about all kinds of things.

That's the effect you want to have on your partner, and also on yourself. You want to get both of your thoughts going, because it's in the head that erotic satisfaction is born. Our bodies may respond to various sensations and physical stimuli, but nothing is as stimulating as the mind—perhaps our most erogenous zone. Once you've engaged it, the body will naturally follow.

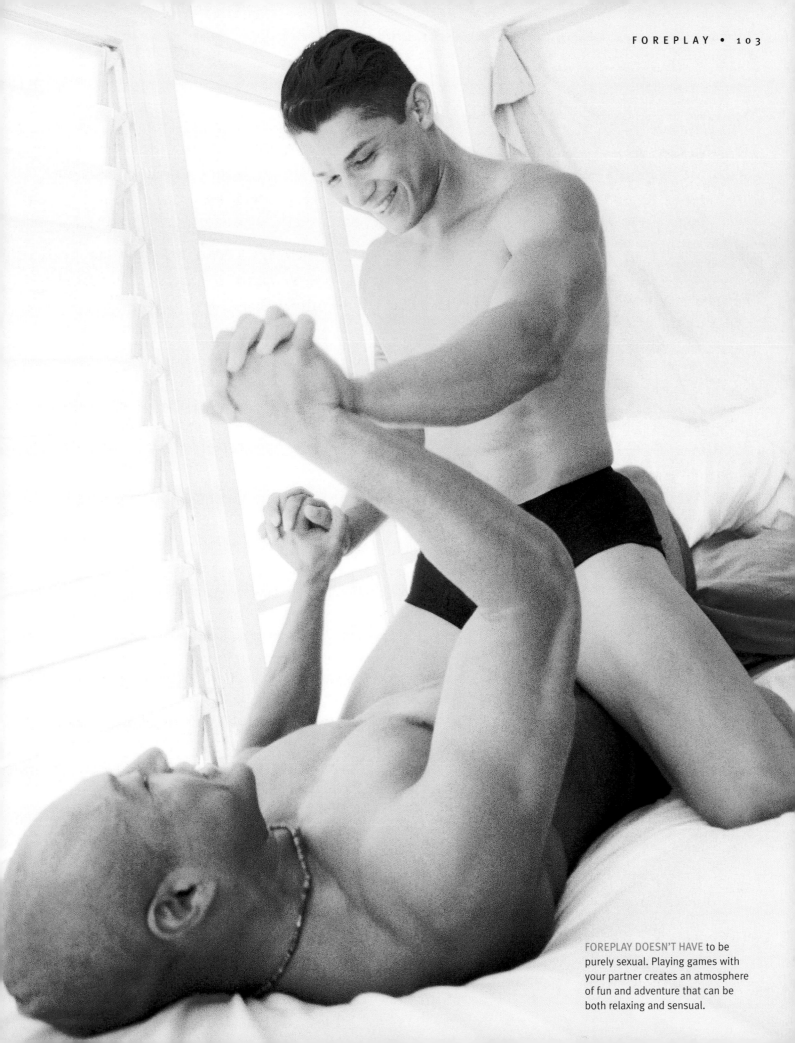

FOREPLAY DOESN'T HAVE to be purely sexual. Playing games with your partner creates an atmosphere of fun and adventure that can be both relaxing and sensual.

Horses for courses

We all find different things sexy and arousing, so what constitutes foreplay for you may be different from what gets your partner all hot and bothered. You may find candlelight and being fed chocolate-covered cherries romantic, while he might prefer having you tie his hands behind his back, put on a jockstrap, and give him an all-over tongue bath. But even if your turn-ons are wildly different, their purpose is the same. You want to get that sexual desire going.

When considering options for foreplay, think about your partner. What does he like? What makes him think about sex? What pushes him to the point where he has to tear your clothes off and throw you on the bed? The possibilities are endless, so don't feel shy about experimenting with different kinds of foreplay; it will pay off!

Does he find competition or being in control arousing? You might try wrestling with him a little bit or teasing him until he (playfully, of course) threatens to put you over his knee and give you a spanking. If he's more the flowers-and-kisses kind of guy, strewing rose petals on

Stages of foreplay

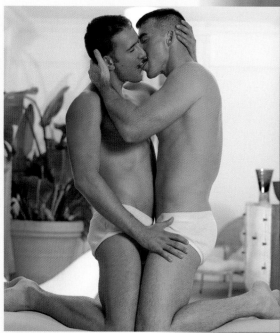

KEEPING YOUR UNDERWEAR on for as long as possible heightens sexual tension by keeping something hidden.

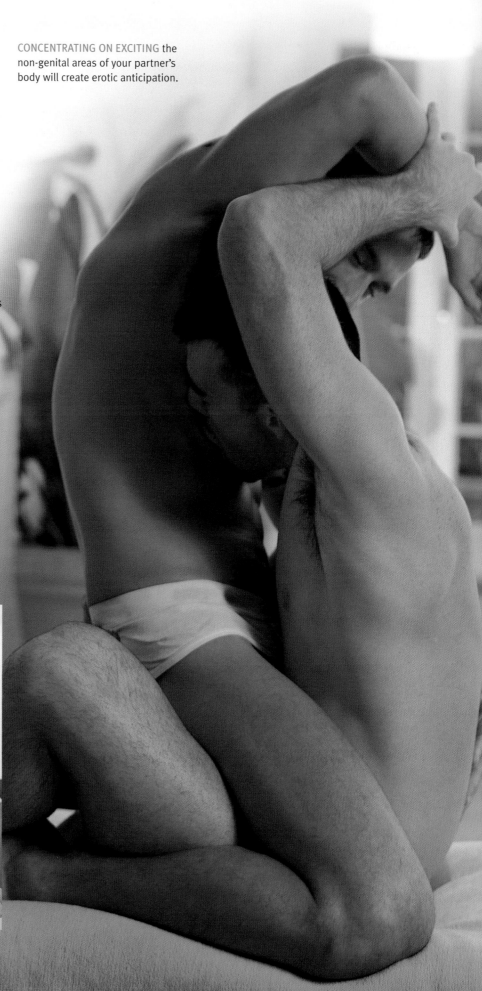

CONCENTRATING ON EXCITING the non-genital areas of your partner's body will create erotic anticipation.

the bed or spending time in a scented bath with him might be a good opening act. Again, it all depends on what he, and you, find exciting.

Time to slow things down

Foreplay doesn't stop once you're in bed, either. In fact, this is where it gets really good. You can create a lot of sexual excitement by taking your time. Don't go right for his penis. Spend some time kissing. Let your hands play over his body. Work him up a little, then slow things down. Don't be in a rush to come. Orgasm should be the by-product of pleasure, and not always the primary goal.

Just as important as arousing your partner is making him comfortable. The more relaxed his body is and the more erotically charged his mind is, the more ready he'll be for making love. Some activities are made much more enjoyable when foreplay is used to put a partner in the mood. For example, spending time touching him and paying attention to his anal area can help ease tensions he might have about anal play. Similarly, touching a partner's body lovingly and letting him know

how exciting you find him can remove fears he might have about body image, making the rest of your time together more fulfilling.

Remember, when it comes to foreplay the mind and the body work together. You want to arouse your partner mentally and stimulate him physically. That means feeding him with ideas (talking dirty, say) while touching him erotically (to find his erogenous zones). When you can combine these two actions, you'll create a sexually charged atmosphere in which anything is possible.

Foreplay is for fun

Foreplay can do wonders for helping an anxious or nervous partner relax and get into the mood for love. If you give him plenty of attention, and take the time to slowly arouse his senses, he'll feel much more comfortable about having sex. He may even show you a trick or two!

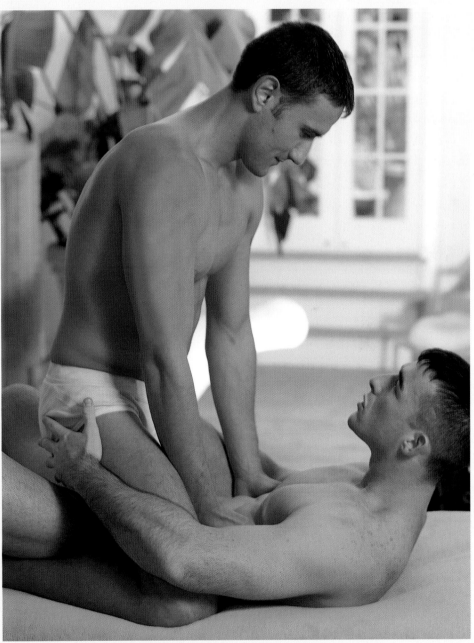

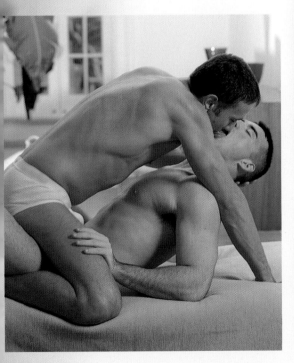

PUSH THINGS FURTHER by being more aggressive and taking erotic play to the next level.

COMMUNICATING WITH YOUR partner and letting him know how excited you are about being with him and how good he makes you feel will get both of you in the mood for more.

Masturbation

A touching experience

For many of us, the first sexual act we ever experience is masturbation. Playing with ourselves seems to come naturally, and even very young boys frequently stimulate themselves manually simply because they have discovered that it feels good. Unfortunately, as we grow older we sometimes come to see masturbation as something to resort to when we can't get "the real thing." This is too bad, because jerking off can be a fantastic way to explore our sexuality, alone or with a partner. What's more it's a really safe way of having sex.

Maximizing pleasure

Masturbation is the act of manually stimulating ourselves or someone else, usually to orgasm, as a way of experiencing sexual pleasure. Sometimes jacking off is simply about releasing sexual tension, while at other times it's a way to explore sexual fantasies or to enhance sexual activities with a partner or partners.

Let's look at solo masturbation first. There are two kinds of men: those who admit they masturbate and those who lie about it. It truly is one of those things that everyone does. How often, and why, is a different story. But I can

guarantee you will never shake a guy's hand that hasn't been responsible for getting him off. We jerk off for a lot of reasons. Often it's because for one reason or another we're not involved with anyone and masturbating is our main sexual outlet. But even when we're involved in relationships or enjoying active sex lives as single men, a lot of us still do it, possibly because we enjoy getting off more frequently than our partners do.

Will I go blind?

We've all heard the old warnings about jerking off: you'll go blind, you'll grow hair on your palms, you'll use up all your semen. We know these "dangers" aren't true. But *is* it possible to masturbate too much? The answer is yes. But it's not because anything unpleasant will happen to you physically; it's because you can actually become addicted to getting yourself off. This occurs when masturbation becomes an obsession, when it totally replaces sexual contact with other men, or when it interferes with your ability to enjoy sex with a partner. Masturbation should be a constituent of a healthy sex life—not your *entire* sex life. If you find that jacking off is the only way you can or want to experience sex, it may be time to see a therapist.

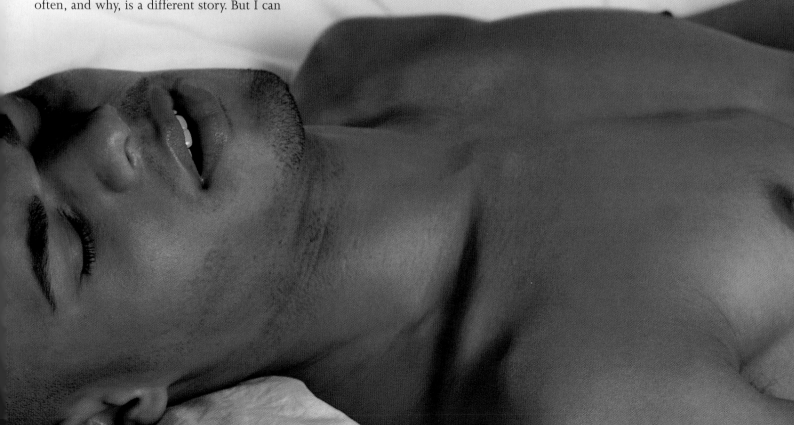

IT HELPS INCREASE the enjoyment of masturbation if you create a pleasurable environment for yourself. Temperature, lighting, and even sound and smell can affect the experience.

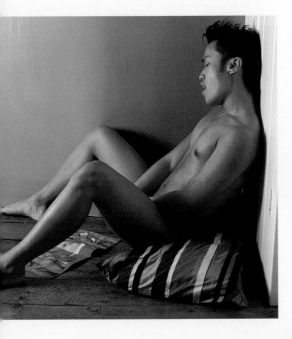

STIMULATING YOURSELF VISUALLY and mentally by looking at erotic images or by fantasizing about different sexual scenarios will create additional excitement and enhance the experience of pleasuring yourself.

you let yourself imagine all kinds of things you want to do and who you want to do them with. We can make love to the actor who makes us crazy, or the guy down the street, or the captain of our favorite hockey team. We can do it with the plumber on the kitchen floor, the fireman on top of the truck, and the road-crew worker right there in the construction zone, while people drive by and honk. We can do it with anyone, anywhere, at any time.

Whatever our reasons for taking matters into our own hands, the beauty of it is that it allows us time to think about what turns us on. Sure, you can come simply from the physical stimulation of the penis. But the best fun is in your head. That's where the real action plays out, where

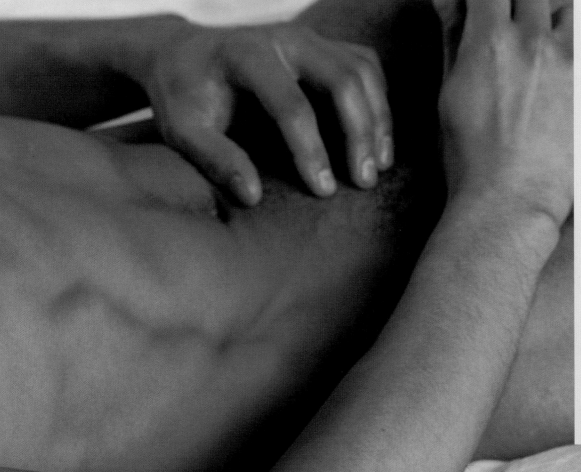

Handy hints

There's no wrong way to masturbate, so try different techniques and see what you like. Some guys like to lubricate their penis when jacking off, while others enjoy it dry. Some use a fast hand motion, others prefer it slow and sensual. This is definitely one activity where practice makes perfect, so experiment with various strokes, positions, and methods of stimulation to see what works for you and what doesn't.

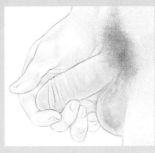

GENTLY FONDLE YOUR flaccid penis. Using lubrication will ensure comfort, particularly if you are circumcised.

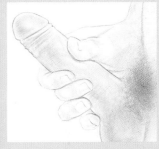

AS YOUR PENIS stiffens, slowly slip your hand up and down the shaft. Repeat this several times.

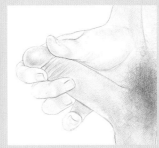

START TO STIMULATE the head. Grasp the penis on the ridge that encircles the tip, and move the skin backward and forward. Then hold the shaft of the penis and stimulate until climax.

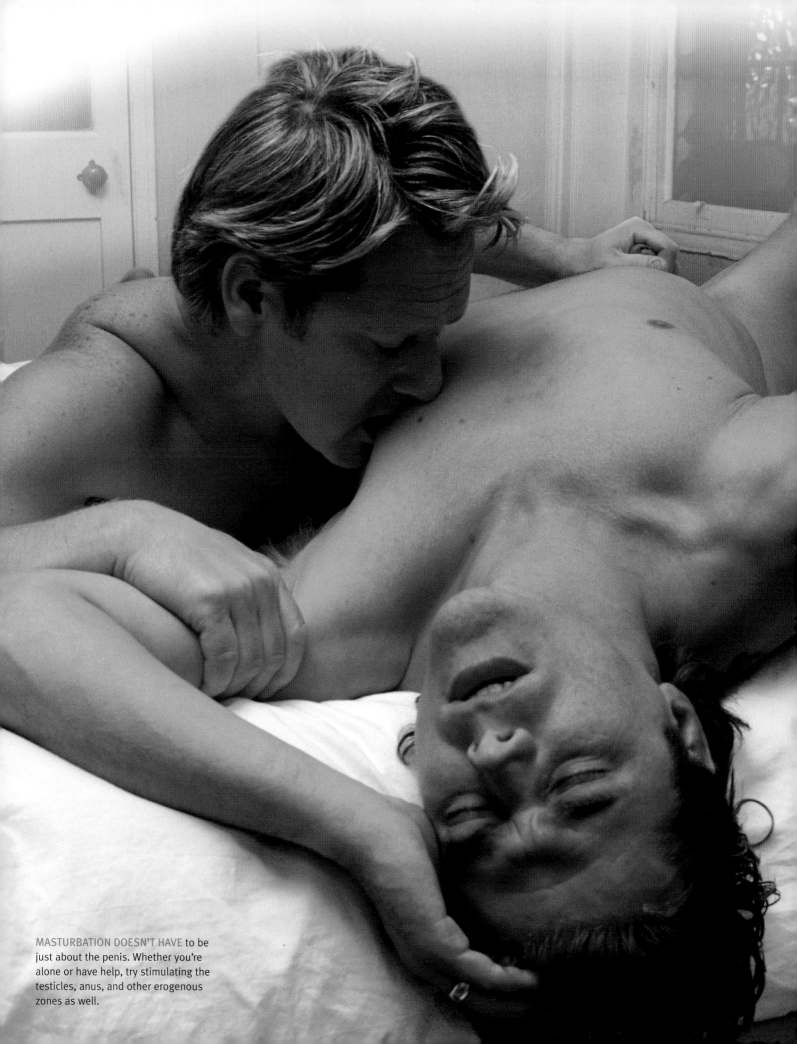

MASTURBATION DOESN'T HAVE to be just about the penis. Whether you're alone or have help, try stimulating the testicles, anus, and other erogenous zones as well.

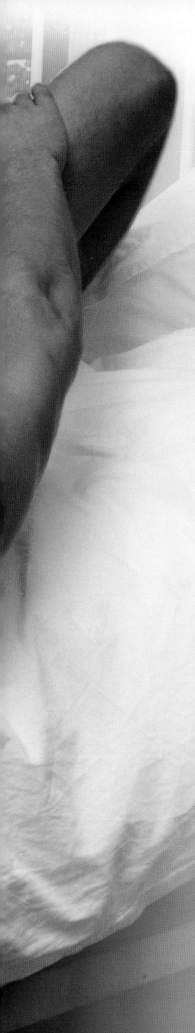

Or perhaps we just want to fantasize about doing different things that we might be interested in but are hesitant to try in real life. Maybe we want to think about being tied up and spanked, or indulging in a three-way, or having our balls shaved. Anything we want to try can safely be done in our fantasies, and seeing how we respond to thinking about these things can be an excellent way to explore our sexual interests.

I'm not telling you to make masturbation a substitute for sex. I'm saying that you should use it as a way to expand your sex life, to see if maybe there are things you're interested in sexually that you haven't yet explored. It's also a way to experience things you might be interested in but can't actually participate in because they aren't available or because your partner isn't interested in them and exploring them outside the relationship is not an option.

As exciting as jacking off is, it *can* become more of a routine than it should be. If playing with yourself has gotten to be as thrilling as brushing your teeth, or if it's something you feel you have to do simply because you can, it's time to liven things up a bit.

Variety is the spice of life

The first thing you need to do is change your routine. If you're jerking off every night before you go to bed, stop. Do it in the morning or when you get home from work. If you tend to always do it in the shower, start doing it on the couch in the living room or in the men's room at the office. Change when and where you do it, and you will make it seem fun again.

You can also try changing what you use for stimulation. If you've been whacking off looking at porn magazines, put them away and try using your own fantasies. If your fantasies have primarily focused on an ex, a movie star, or even a politician, try picking another erotic focus. And if you're tired of your own fantasies, try watching an erotic movie and jerking off along with the guys on the screen.

There are so many ways we can arouse ourselves: words, pictures, sounds, smells. Use all of them. Create an environment that adds to the fun and excitement of masturbating. If you enjoy getting off in your bedroom, make your bed an inviting place to be. The sheets on the bed, the lights or candles that illuminate the space, the smell of incense or flowers—all of these things can add to the experience.

Setting the scene gets you off to a good start by helping you get into the experience. Say, for example, you like to fantasize about getting off with a mechanic. There's nothing that says you can't go into your garage, lean up against a workbench, and whack off, surrounded by tools

It's not taboo anymore

The history of masturbation goes back a long way, probably well before the Egyptians, who believed that the Nile River rose each year because of the continuous masturbation of the god Osiris. His sperm was said to be the source of all living things. From this grand vision, the concept of masturbation has taken a downturn over the centuries, especially in Western cultures, where it has been deemed immoral, dirty, a taboo, and even a symptom of disease or madness. Thankfully, these days, far less social stigma is attached to an activity men have always enjoyed. So, in the spirit of the first advocates and celebrants of masturbation, go ahead, relish each part of your own—and your partner's—body. The idea is to give each other as much pleasure as you can. Start by getting naked, then slowly and sensually begin to discover each sexy, delicious spot, from the top of your partner's head all the way down to his toes.

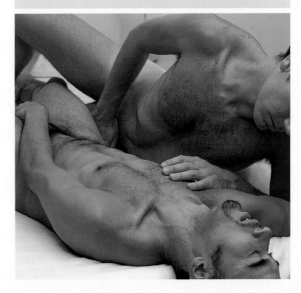

• Try experimenting with different sensations. If you wrap a piece of silk, leather, or fur around your shaft (or your partner's) when masturbating, it will create a fantastically different feeling.

• Try using a hand-held massager or vibrator to stimulate the genitals. Or experiment with a shower massager: Maybe you can bring yourself to orgasm by passing it along your shaft.

• Incorporate items such as jockstraps or underwear into your masturbation play, using them to jerk off with or to smell or taste while getting off.

• Creams and sprays used to delay orgasm can also allow you to extend the length of time that you can hold off on coming while you masturbate. Experiment with one.

• Masturbating while wearing a condom can create a pleasurable sensation, and some guys get off on seeing themselves shoot into a rubber.

• Wearing a cock ring while jacking off can add additional physical and visual stimulation.

and the smell of oil. Or if being outdoors stirs your imagination, find a secluded spot in the woods, on a beach, or on a mountaintop.

Keep in mind that all these ideas work whether you're jacking off alone or with a partner. The goal is to make masturbating an activity that's just as fulfilling as any other sexual act. Instead of treating self-love as a backup, elevate it to another level. Use it both as a way to get off and as a doorway that can lead you to an exploration of other aspects of your sexuality.

Playing with a partner

Masturbation is usually thought of as something we do alone. But it can also be an important part of sex with a partner, or several partners. For one thing, it's a very safe activity, with almost no possibility for transmission of STDs. This makes it a perfect way to play with someone you don't want to be more intimate with.

It can also be a great way to explore each other's bodies and find out what kind of stimulation you both like. When you play with a partner's penis, you find out how he likes it to be held, stroked, squeezed, and otherwise touched. It also allows you to pay attention

to other body parts or activities at the same time. You can kiss while stroking each other, for example, or incorporate masturbation into massage or frottage.

Some couples use jerking off in addition to oral and anal sex. One partner may masturbate while being anally penetrated, for example, or might jack off while blowing the other. Partners may like to pleasure themselves while looking at, and enjoying, each other's bodies.

When playing with a partner, experiment with ways you can use masturbation in your lovemaking. Sit facing each other and jerk each other off. Straddle your partner while he's on his back and hold your penises together, stroking them with one hand as

Mutual masturbation

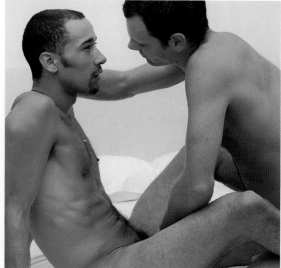

WHEN JERKING OFF with a partner, pay attention to how he responds to different types of touch. Change your strokes and grip to create the greatest level of excitement.

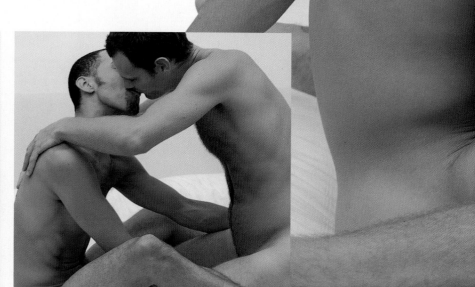

INCLUDING MASTURBATION with other activities, such as kissing, creates another layer of erotic sensation and adds to the experience of making love with a partner.

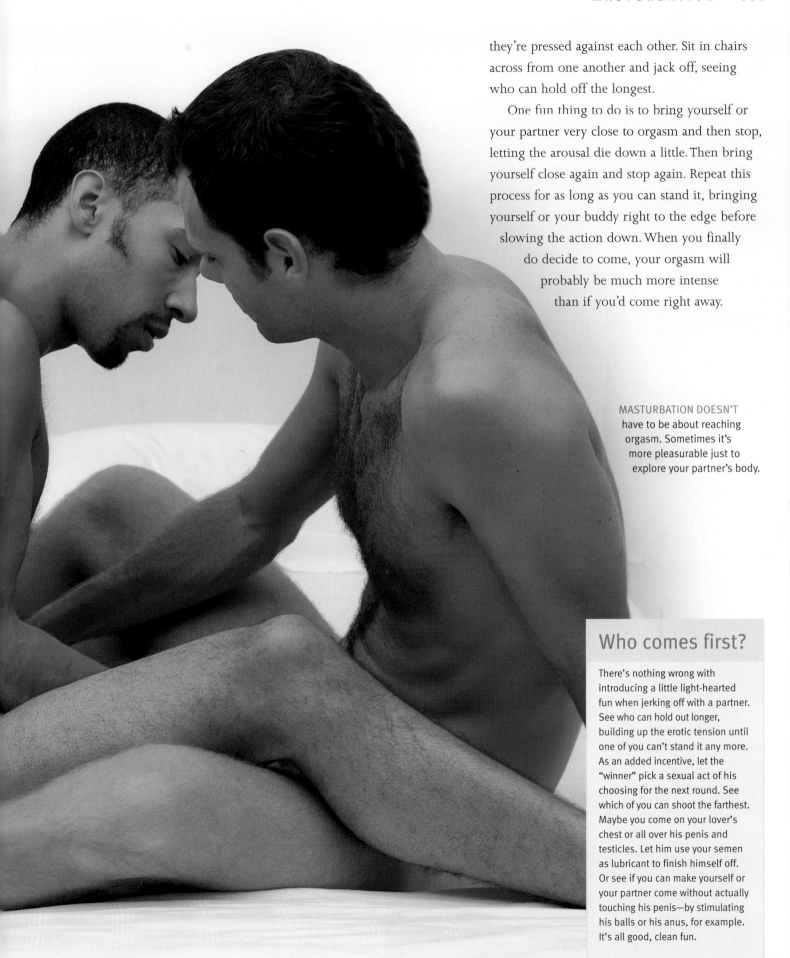

they're pressed against each other. Sit in chairs across from one another and jack off, seeing who can hold off the longest.

One fun thing to do is to bring yourself or your partner very close to orgasm and then stop, letting the arousal die down a little. Then bring yourself close again and stop again. Repeat this process for as long as you can stand it, bringing yourself or your buddy right to the edge before slowing the action down. When you finally do decide to come, your orgasm will probably be much more intense than if you'd come right away.

MASTURBATION DOESN'T have to be about reaching orgasm. Sometimes it's more pleasurable just to explore your partner's body.

Who comes first?

There's nothing wrong with introducing a little light-hearted fun when jerking off with a partner. See who can hold out longer, building up the erotic tension until one of you can't stand it any more. As an added incentive, let the "winner" pick a sexual act of his choosing for the next round. See which of you can shoot the farthest. Maybe you come on your lover's chest or all over his penis and testicles. Let him use your semen as lubricant to finish himself off. Or see if you can make yourself or your partner come without actually touching his penis—by stimulating his balls or his anus, for example. It's all good, clean fun.

Frottage

Never too close for comfort

Frottage (pronounced "fro-TAJ") is simply a fancy French word for dry humping. The term is actually derived from an art technique, but in sexual parlance it refers to exciting yourself by rubbing your genitals up against something or, more often, someone. In the strictest definition you would do this while clothed, but we're not all that strict around here so we're using it to mean rubbing up against someone while clothed or naked.

The origins of frottage

With its French origins and sophisticated sound, you'd think frottage might be some exotic activity created by courtesans in Paris. Really it was pretty much invented by horny teenagers in the back seats of cars, or maybe carriages way back when. For many people inhibited by social or religious rules, rubbing up against one another was as good as it got. Afraid or unable to shed their clothes and go at it, they settled for the next best thing.

Oh, but how we've progressed. Now we know that frottage has all kinds of erotic possibilities, and it's climbed out of the back seat and become an integral part of lovemaking. No more the fallback plan for frustrated lovers, it's a pleasure unto itself, and experimenting with the joys it brings will make your own sex life that much better.

Getting a feel for things

Because it retains some aspects of forbidden sex, frottage can be a real turn-on. Rubbing yourself against a partner, particularly when still dressed, provides the promise of sex to come. Feeling a lover's hard penis pressed against you through his jeans or underwear but not seeing it or touching it directly makes you think about what it will look, feel, and taste like. It starts a fantasy in your mind about what you might be doing once the clothes do come off.

Once the clothes *are* off, frottage provides the experience of feeling a partner's body against our own. The way his muscles move, how his chest hair

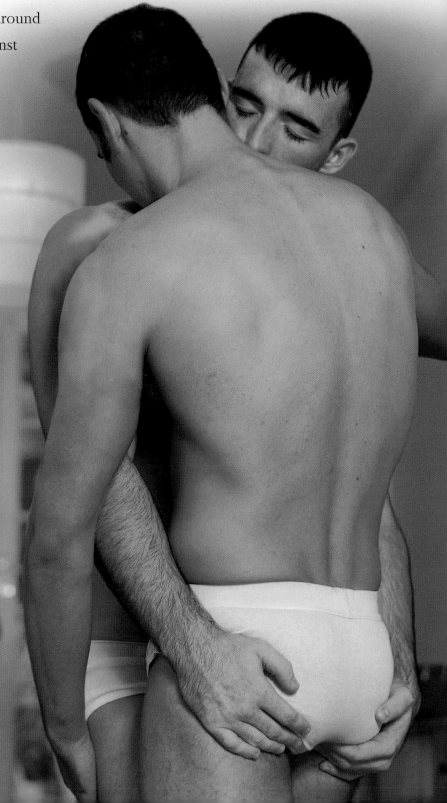

KEEPING YOUR UNDERWEAR on can be just as sexy as taking it off. See if you can make your lover come by stimulating him through his shorts.

feels sliding across your bare back, the touch of his penis slipping between your butt cheeks—these extremely erotic sensations can only fuel your passion. Simply being covered by another man's body, having him hold you while thrusting against you, can be intensely arousing.

Orgasm might or might not be the desired result of this activity. Some guys like to come while rubbing against a partner, perhaps while

grinding against each other face to face, or by simulating anal sex by placing the penis between the butt cheeks or legs and thrusting. But for others, frottage is a way to heighten the rest of the action. However you enjoy it, pay attention to how your body is interacting with your lover's. Move deliberately, sliding a hand here, pressing him there, and feel how all these different sensations add to the experience.

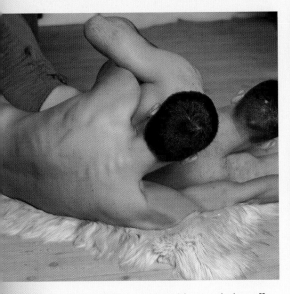

Lying down positions

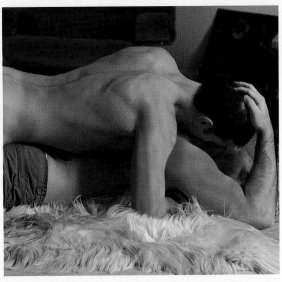

MOST OF THE POSITIONS you enjoy with your clothes off can also be enjoyed with your clothes on. See how different, yet equally erotic, they feel clothed and unclothed.

THE CONTRASTING FEELINGS of skin against clothing is what makes frottage so exciting for some people. Different fabrics and materials can create different sensations.

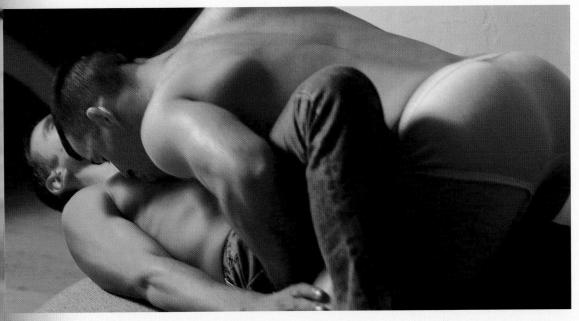

IF RUBBING AGAINST someone's clothed body gets you off, have your partner keep his jeans on while you simulate

making love to him. Non-penetrative sex doesn't mean unenjoyable sex.

Keeping covered

Don't immediately strip down when you're ready to get it on with a partner. Draw out the experience by spending some time with your clothes on. Let your hands move over his clothed body and imagine what it looks like beneath his business suit or T-shirt and jeans. Put your hand between his legs and give him a squeeze, feeling how his penis strains against the material. Press yourself against him so he can feel how aroused he's making you.

When you're ready to take things a step further, unzip or unbutton his pants and slide your hand inside, gripping his penis through his underwear and giving it a squeeze. Unbutton or remove his shirt and straddle him, pressing yourself against his bare skin.

Vary the motion and pressure of your thrusting, using circular motions as well as back-and-forth movements. Friction resulting from frottage can be painful—often only surfacing a while after the event.

Use the time before you're completely naked to tease your partner—and to heighten expectations. Enjoy the feeling of knowing that beneath his clothes there's something really exciting waiting for you. Whether you're with a new partner or a long-time love, you can make this experience a powerful one if you focus on how stimulating the feel of clothed bodies against one another, or against bare skin, can be.

Standing positions

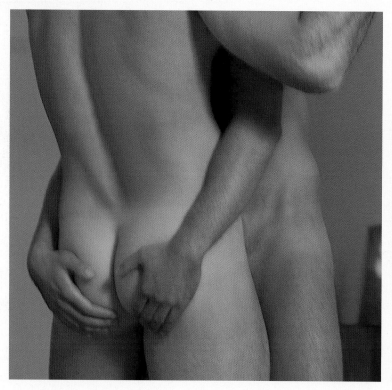

GRABBING THE CHEEKS of your partner's ass, press your erect penis against his, thrusting up with your hips to create friction. Synchronize your thrusting movements to double your pleasure.

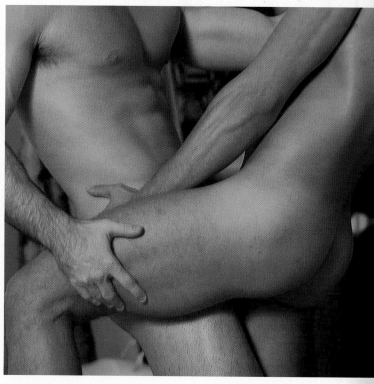

STRADDLING YOUR PARTNER'S leg and rubbing your genitals against it can create a pleasurable physical and visual stimulation for both of you. Making occasional eye contact while doing so can be intensely erotic.

Frottage fun

Want to try a little frottage but aren't sure how to introduce it to your partner? Use one of these scenarios as a jumping-off point.

• Buy yourself or your partner some new underwear, something sexy like boxer briefs or silk shorts.

• Get home before your partner does and strip down. When he walks in the door, have him sit on the couch while you straddle him.

• Stage a wrestling match—clothed or unclothed—with your partner. Don't worry about who wins, just enjoy the body-on-body action.

• Using handcuffs, rope, or even neckties, secure your partner's hands and try to get him off just by rubbing your body against his.

• The next time you're in an elevator, get behind your partner and press up against him. If you can do it while hard, all the better.

There's the rub

For some people the appeal of frottage lies in the combination of seeing and feeling different types of clothing against the skin. If, for example, you find the feel of leather a turn-on, you might get off on the idea of rubbing up against someone dressed in leather pants or a leather jacket. If the sight of a guy in a jockstrap appeals to you, having your partner (or both of you) wear one and pressing against one another might be arousing.

Similarly, it could be exciting for you to strip down, while your lover keeps on his business suit, work clothes, or even his sweaty gym shorts. Grinding against him or having him rub against your naked body while dressed this way could be part of a larger fantasy. Many men like the idea of ejaculating on someone's clothes, so if this appeals to you use it as part of your frottage fun.

Speaking of fantasy, the idea of frottage appeals to some men because of its association with forbidden sex. They may like the idea

of pressing up against someone on a subway car or in an elevator, for example, or of having someone press up against them. They might become aroused by the thought of someone unexpectedly putting a hand between their legs while sitting beside them in an airplane or in some other public place. You can incorporate these kinds of fantasies into your sex life, either by actually engaging in them with a partner, when possible, or by simulating them in private.

The power of touch

Ultimately, frottage involves a combination of sensations, whether it's skin on skin, clothes on clothes, or skin on clothes. Frottage is also about setting and situation, fantasy and fetish. When these elements combine, the experience can be wonderfully erotic, so use your imagination and see what a little bumping and grinding can do for your sex life.

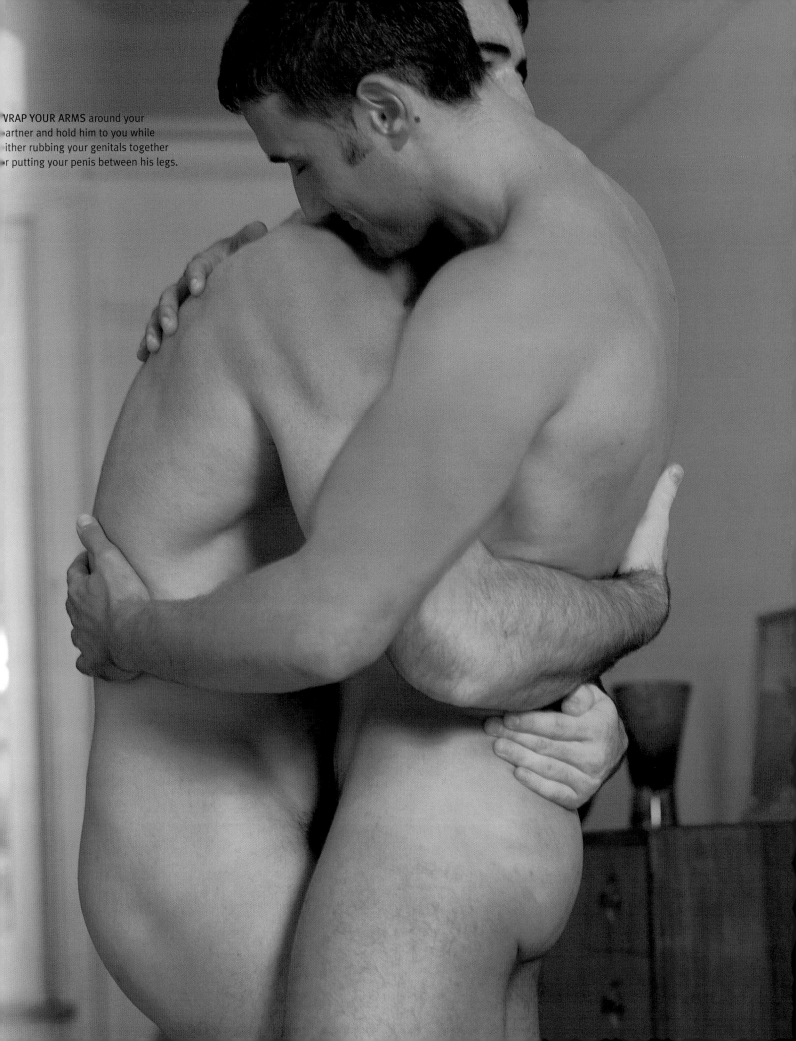

WRAP YOUR ARMS around your
partner and hold him to you while
either rubbing your genitals together
or putting your penis between his legs.

Oral sex

Exploring the art

A straight male friend of mine once said, "There's no such thing as a bad blow job." This is simply not true. There are horrible blow jobs, mediocre blow jobs, and, thankfully, there are incredible blow jobs. What makes a blow job bad, good, or amazing is partially a matter of what the lucky fellow receiving it likes. But there are also some basic skills involved in doing it right, and knowing these skills and how to perform them expertly will virtually guarantee that those fortunate enough to experience your techniques will come again, perhaps in more ways than one.

Paying lip service

Although my friend who said that there's no such thing as a bad blow job wasn't entirely accurate, it's true that most men won't object to a little oral action. In fact, for many men it's about the best thing that can happen to them on any given day (or on any given date). A good blow job, performed with skill and enthusiasm, is right up there with having your favorite team win the World Series or your favorite actress take home the Oscar. Okay, it's a lot better than those things. It's like hitting the home run that wins the Series for your team. The point is, blow jobs are a whole lotta fun and we love receiving them.

What is it about putting your penis in someone's mouth or having someone's penis in your mouth that's so arousing? Like kissing, oral sex is a form of intercourse in miniature. Also, there's something a little forbidden about it. As children, many of us are taught that our genitals are off-limits. Well, what could be more rebellious than putting someone's naughty bits in our mouth, or ours in his? This element of taboo makes it all just that much more exciting.

Going down?

The truth is, oral sex is all about worshipping the penis and, to a lesser degree, the guy it belongs to. Let's just admit that right up front. And so what? The penis is a really, really cool thing, and why shouldn't we give it some attention now and then? If you're the one who's giving the blow job, you're in effect celebrating the joys of the penis. Taking it into your mouth, sucking it, licking it, tasting it, and fondling it are all ways of enjoying what the penis is and what it can do.

Giving head is, on some level, a way of submitting to your partner, of becoming responsible for his pleasure. But it's also an act of power. You have one of the most precious and sensitive parts of your partner's body in your mouth. You're controlling his enjoyment with your actions. Many men enjoy assuming this role, and for some guys the sense of power they feel from giving head is more fulfilling than other forms of sexual activity.

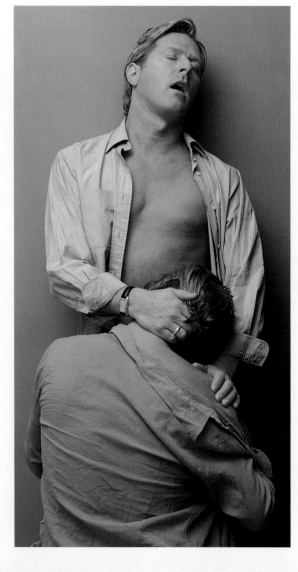

PERFORMING ORAL SEX on your partner is one of the most intimate sexual gifts you can give him. Adding a few words of appreciation for how his penis feels in your mouth will make him smile all the more.

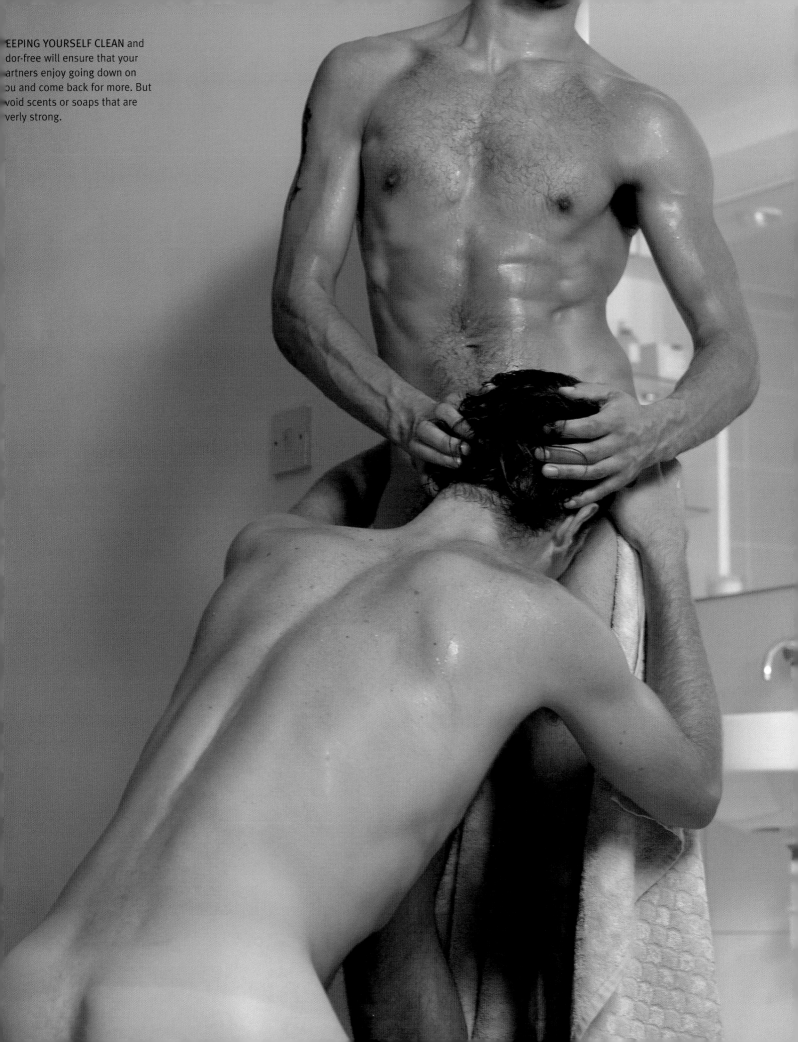

EEPING YOURSELF CLEAN and
dor-free will ensure that your
artners enjoy going down on
ou and come back for more. But
void scents or soaps that are
verly strong.

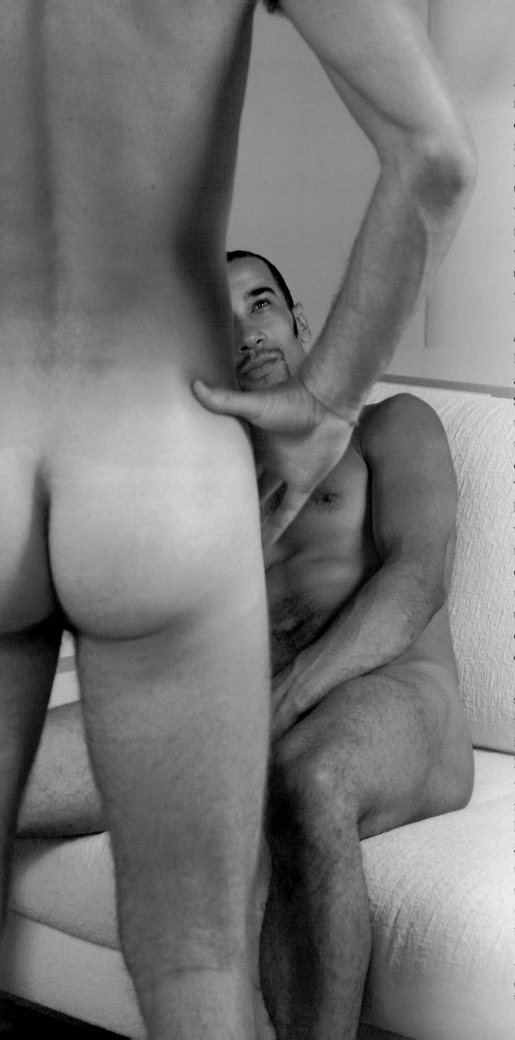

As the guy receiving the blow job, you
may feel you're exerting some form of
dominance over your partner, particularly
if you're directing the action physically or with
your words. This can add to the excitement of
the act. You may also get off on the fact that
your penis is being enjoyed by this man who
finds you and your penis arousing enough to
want to pay attention to you. And let's not forget
that the pure physical sensations of having
your penis sucked are incredibly enjoyable.

A time and a place

Like any sexual act, oral sex shouldn't simply be
about getting in there and getting the job done.
Sure, sometimes all we want is the blow job. But
usually it's part of a larger plan, a way to build
up excitement before other activities or a means
of bringing lovemaking to a dramatic close.
There's no rule that says giving head has to
happen at a particular time or in a particular
way. Some guys like to use it as foreplay before
moving on to other forms of stimulation, while
others enjoy finishing off a session of anal sex by
using oral sex to reach orgasm. And, of course,
there are many other possibilities for introducing
oral action into sexual play. When and how you
do it is entirely up to you and your partners.

At whatever point you decide to do it, you
should approach giving head in the same way
you would approach stimulating your partner
in any other way. Start by building anticipation.
Don't dive for the penis right away. You want
your lover to think about how you're going to
make him feel, since this will raise his excitement
level. Start, perhaps, by kissing or licking the area
around his penis. Play with his testicles, and
tease him a little. When it's time to move to
the penis itself, gently lick the head or run
your tongue along the shaft. Then slide the head
between your lips, letting it rest there while you

THE ENJOYMENT OF ORAL sex begins before your mouth
even touches his penis. Let him know that you're going
to make him feel good and that you'll enjoy doing it.

Should he come in my mouth?

Whether or not to let a partner ejaculate in your mouth is one of the biggest issues about oral sex. The decision is partly a matter of preference. Some guys like the taste of semen and some don't. Some find the idea of a guy coming in their mouth a real turn-on, while others find the whole business highly unpleasant. Safety is another issue. HIV can be transmitted through cuts in the mouth, and although incidents of infection via oral sex are thought to be very rare, some men don't want to expose themselves to even the slightest risk. Whether you do or don't allow your partner to ejaculate in your mouth (swallowing afterward is not really the issue) is ultimately a personal decision that should be based on understanding the possible risks involved, and on what you find sexually exciting.

tongue it. If your partner wants to control the action by telling you what to do, by thrusting his hips, or by using his hands on your head, let him (unless it's uncomfortable for you). This control may form a large part of his enjoyment.

It's the way that you do it

Your technique is going to depend partly on what you like and partly on what your partner likes. Some guys enjoy taking the full length of a partner's penis into their mouth or throat. For some men this is uncomfortable or it may even be impossible, particularly if a lover's penis is

HOW YOU POSITION yourself for oral sex can increase the enjoyment of the activity. Kneeling between his legs may give him a sense of power he finds arousing.

very thick or long. Simply do what's comfortable for you. (If you find that your instinct is to gag from the sensation of feeling your partner's penis in your throat, you can usually overcome this by relaxing and breathing through your nose rather than your mouth.)

If getting your partner's penis into your mouth is difficult, you can always concentrate on the head, especially if you stroke and pump the shaft with your hand at the same time. Use your tongue to trace the contours of his penis, moving from the head to the balls and back again. Running the tip of your tongue around

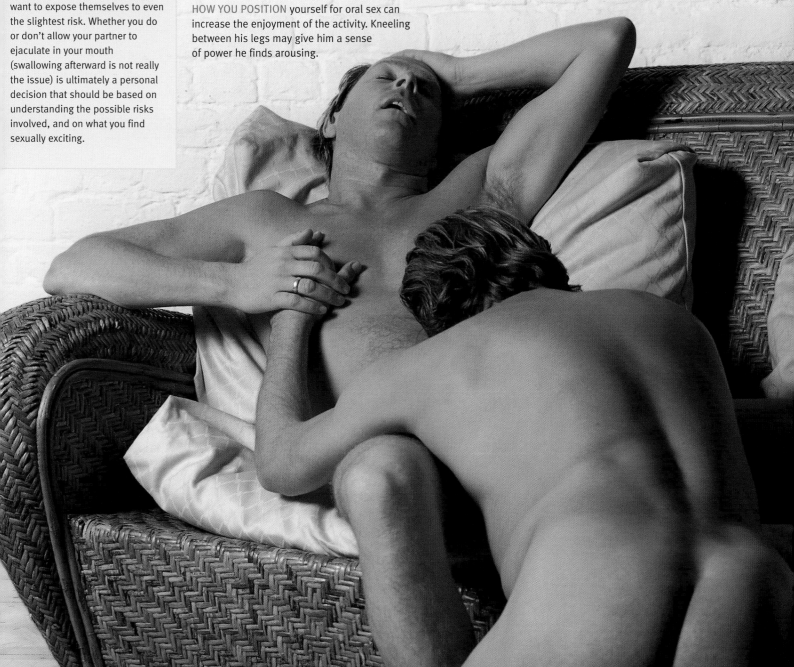

the ridge of the head will be a particular turn-on. Or give him an unusual sensation by gently nibbling the side of his penis. If you can get most of his penis in, moving your mouth up and down may be the way to go. You can also try very gently drawing his balls (usually one at a time) into your mouth and suck on them. Again, it all depends on what feels good to you and your partner. Whatever technique you use in oral sex, the important thing is that you focus on making it pleasurable. Sure, you can make a guy come just by stroking him or licking his penis, but why not really get into it? Why not make it an experience you both enjoy and one which makes whatever else you do together that much more fun.

Knowing what you like best

Think of oral sex as a way of celebrating everything you love about the penis and about making love with men. And when you've got another guy's penis in your mouth, think too about what makes you feel good when it

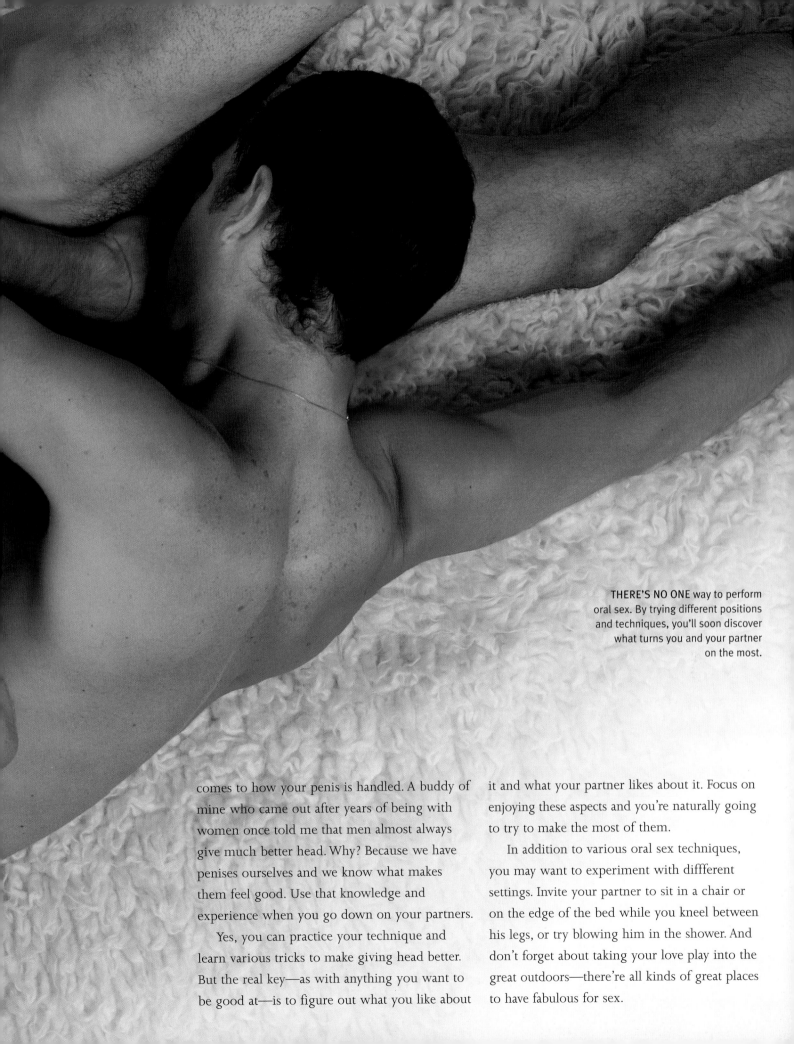

THERE'S NO ONE way to perform oral sex. By trying different positions and techniques, you'll soon discover what turns you and your partner on the most.

comes to how your penis is handled. A buddy of mine who came out after years of being with women once told me that men almost always give much better head. Why? Because we have penises ourselves and we know what makes them feel good. Use that knowledge and experience when you go down on your partners.

Yes, you can practice your technique and learn various tricks to make giving head better. But the real key—as with anything you want to be good at—is to figure out what you like about

it and what your partner likes about it. Focus on enjoying these aspects and you're naturally going to try to make the most of them.

In addition to various oral sex techniques, you may want to experiment with diffferent settings. Invite your partner to sit in a chair or on the edge of the bed while you kneel between his legs, or try blowing him in the shower. And don't forget about taking your love play into the great outdoors—there're all kinds of great places to have fabulous for sex.

Anal sex

The ins and outs

When I was dispensing sex advice in the pages of men's magazines, the topic I received the most mail about was anal sex: how to do it, how to keep it clean, how to make sure it didn't hurt. It became clear very early on that for many men, anal sex was a complete mystery, one they weren't quite sure how to go about unraveling. Well, here's some good news. Anal sex does *not* have to hurt, is relatively easy to figure out, and will bring you a whole lot of enjoyment once you do. It just takes a little patience, practice, and lots and lots of lube.

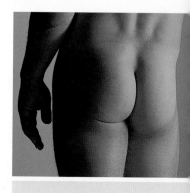

Anatomy lesson

The anus is the opening to the rectum, which is the end of the large intestine. The opening and closing of the anus is the work of the sphincter, a ring of muscle that expands and contracts. Most often, pain associated with anal sex is experienced in this area, when you try to force the sphincter to open before it's ready.

This is where experimentation can help. By playing with your anus and seeing how your sphincter responds to different stimuli, you can learn to relax during anal sex and determine what kind of stimulation you need before your partner inserts his penis.

The basics

We'll get into some fun stuff involving different positions for anal sex in a little bit. But first let's get into the basics. For starters, why would anyone want to have anal sex? I'll tell you why—because when it's done right it feels great. The rectum is a very sensitive part of the body. In addition, the prostate responds incredibly well to stimulation, and anal sex is great for giving it a little attention. In addition, the psychological satisfaction gained from making love with a partner this way adds enormously to the physical pleasure. The number one reason men don't enjoy anal sex or think they can't have anal sex is pain—either real or imagined. Maybe they've tried sticking a finger up there and can't even imagine how something bigger would find its

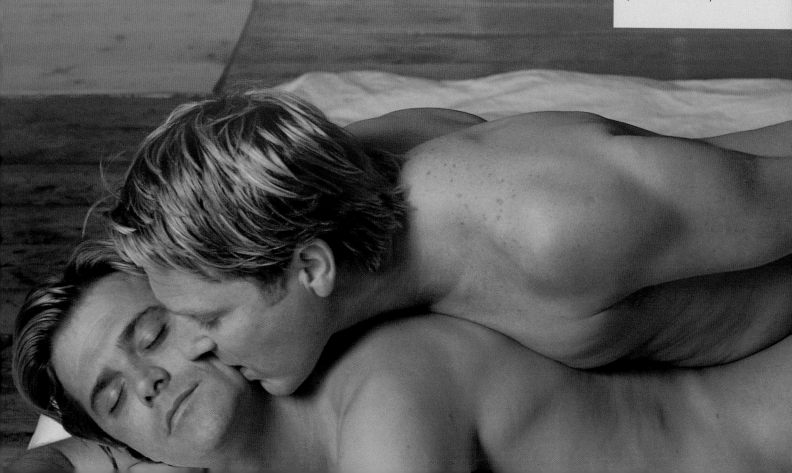

way inside. Perhaps they've actually had a penis in there and found it so painful they couldn't enjoy it. Or maybe the fear is completely anticipatory, with no first-hand experience to back it up. Well, repeat after me: Anal sex does not have to hurt. And the key to making it not hurt are those three things I mentioned earlier: relaxation, patience, and plenty of lubrication. Let's look at these elements in a little more detail.

Relax those muscles

The sphincter is a ring of muscle designed to open and shut like the futuristic doors you see on spaceships in movies. In order for anal sex to be pain-free, that doorway has to be coaxed open. You do this by relaxing the sphincter muscles, but first, you need to relax your whole body. If you're tense, you're going to freeze up as soon as your partner gets anywhere near your

WITH A LITTLE patience and practice, anal sex can be an intensely pleasurable activity for both partners, encompassing a wide range of sensations.

butt. So settle down. Second, have him stimulate your anus with his fingers, his tongue, or whatever tickles your fanny, er, fancy.

This stimulation helps you relax and gets you a little worked up sexually. Once you're aroused, it's easier to go to the next step. This is where your partner inserts his penis into your bum. Now, your first instinct might be to snap that door shut. But try to relax. Breathe. Even more important, make sure your butt and his penis are slicked up with lots of lube, which will make sliding in and out a lot easier. It will also reduce the unpleasant friction that causes most of the discomfort during anal sex.

Slowing things down

This is where patience comes in. Trust me, if your partner takes his time, you will get that thing in there. But he has to be willing to go at your pace. If he goes in inch by inch, allowing you to adjust to feeling him inside of you, things will be just fine.

Wash & go!

One of the biggest fears about anal sex is that it might get a little dirty down there, but keeping clean is easy. All you have to do is douche. Buy yourself a plain old enema at the drugstore. You can use the solution that comes in it for the first time, and after that you can simply unscrew the cap and fill the plastic bottle with warm (not hot) water. Avoid adding soap, though, as it can dry out the rectum and make scraping or tearing it easier.

Gently insert the tip of the enema into your rectum and squeeze the water inside. Hold it for a moment, then expel it. Repeat as necessary until everything is squeaky clean. Enema bottles are small and compact, and can fit in an overnight bag or even (for the man on the go) a jacket pocket.

If you find yourself in a situation where you don't have your handy enema bottle with you, don't worry, you can give yourself a quick finger check. Simply slide it in, check around for any unwanted cargo, and clean house.

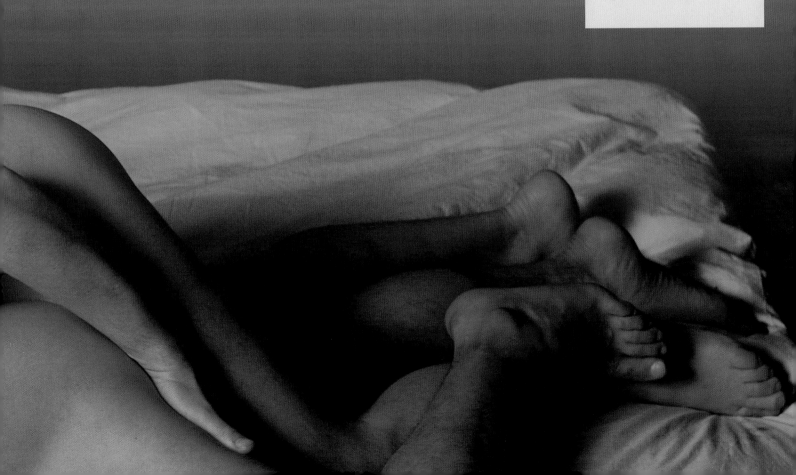

Missionary position
Taking it lying down

This position allows face-to-face contact between partners, making kissing and touching an added bonus. It gives the guy doing the pumping more freedom of movement, and he can achieve deeper penetration by pushing his partner's legs back, which can help in stimulating the prostate. The receptive partner can easily jerk off in this position as well, allowing the partners to come together. And if you want to watch each other shoot, the active partner can slip out when he's close to coming, or you can press your penises together and one or the other of you can do the honors.

Take your positions

Let's take a moment to talk about the whole top/bottom thing. You know, where you only do the fucking or you're the one that only gets fucked. I know a lot of you think you're only one or the other, or that you're only supposed to be one or the other. Well, get over it. Being able to try either activity, and to decide which you prefer, is your free choice. And don't let anyone tell you otherwise. There's nothing wrong with preferring one role to the other, but every guy should at least try both giving and receiving, if only to know what it feels like. When you experience what it's like to be on a particular end of the action, it helps you to know how to make your partner's experience more exciting. So even if it's only once a year that you do it, take turns giving and receiving. It will make you a better lover, and maybe even a better person.

Mission accomplished

In the missionary position it's the top who's in control of the action. That means if you're doing the driving you get to decide when things speed up and when things slow down. How fast and hard you pump your partner's butt will determine how it feels for him, so be conscious of that. Don't just pump away like you're doing push-ups. Vary the force of your strokes and their speed to give him (and you) different sensations. This will go a long way toward making your experience a more pleasurable one.

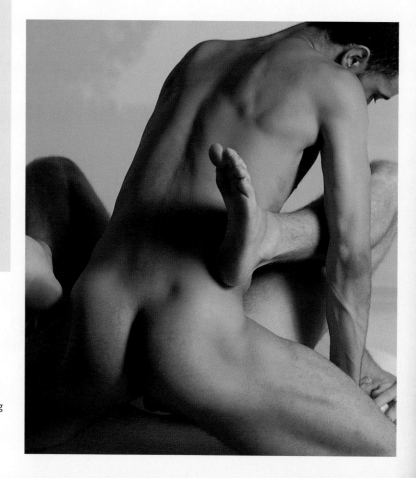

SEX SHOULDN'T BE confined solely to the bed. Use the couch, the stairs, the floor. Experiment with positioning yourselves at various heights and in various ways to see if it creates different sensations.

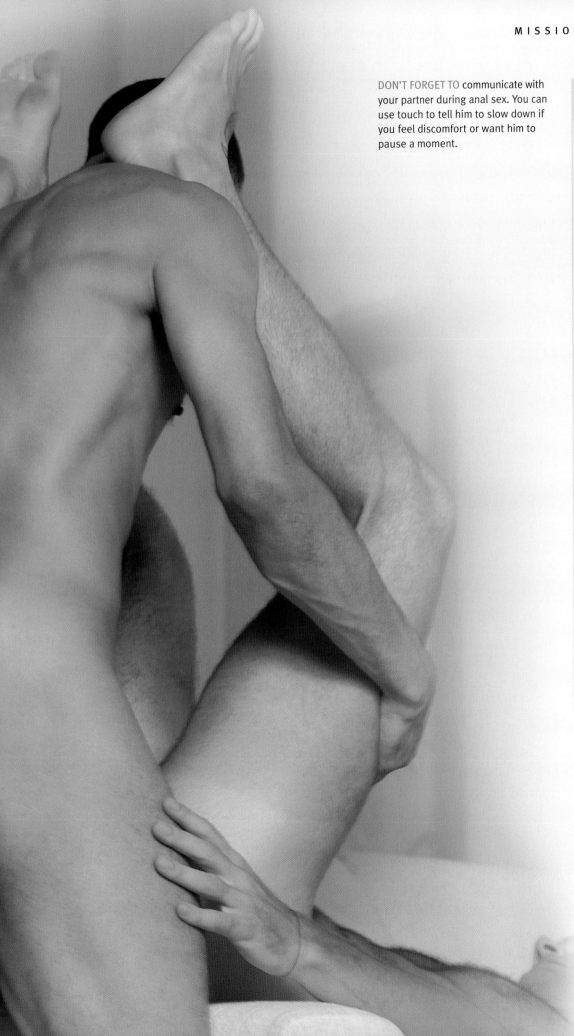

DON'T FORGET TO communicate with your partner during anal sex. You can use touch to tell him to slow down if you feel discomfort or want him to pause a moment.

Are you coming?

Although some men find that they can reach orgasm simply from being fucked, others require manual or oral stimulation, either during or after anal sex, to come. Others find that they actually *can't* come from anal activity.

Whether you can or can't depends on a number of things, including what stimulates you and how your body responds to this stimulation. For many men anal play is incredibly arousing and orgasm occurs as a result. For other men the stimulation (particularly of the prostate) can actually be so intensely pleasurable as to be overwhelming, making it very hard to come without additional activity.

Again, this is going to differ from guy to guy, so knowing how your own body responds to different types of stimulation will help you know what's going on during sex. And remember, orgasm is not always the goal. Not coming from anal sex doesn't mean not enjoying it.

If you find that you or your partner don't reach orgasm during anal sex, incorporate other forms of stimulation into your play to help both of you come. It's often easiest if the top partner comes first and then helps the other partner get off, because getting fucked after coming is sometimes less comfortable for the receptive partner.

Doggie style

A little ruff and tumble

Many men enjoy anal sex from behind (also called doggie style). It can sometimes be more comfortable than face-to-face positions, and it allows for deep, fast, and forceful strokes. The position can work with partners kneeling, standing, or lying down, making it useful in many different situations and for partners of different heights. This position also allows for spanking of the receptive partner's butt, which some men find incredibly arousing. When using the kneeling position, the active partner may grasp the other's shoulders for deeper penetration.

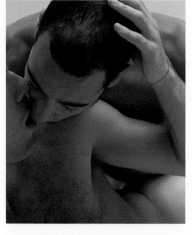

ENTERING YOUR PARTNER while he's on his stomach makes kissing possible and may be more comfortable.

Easier on all fours

Rear-entry positions are particularly good for men who are concerned about pain-related issues. Being on your hands and knees, or lying on your stomach, is often the most comfortable position for both partners, making it easier to relax. This position allows the top to take his time entering the anus, making it easier to pause if necessary to give the bottom time to adjust. In the classic doggie-style position, the angle of insertion can also be changed by having the receptive partner raise or lower his ass to find the most comfortable position. Once the penis is inserted, either partner can control the action, with the bottom moving back and forth along the top's penis or the top doing the pumping.

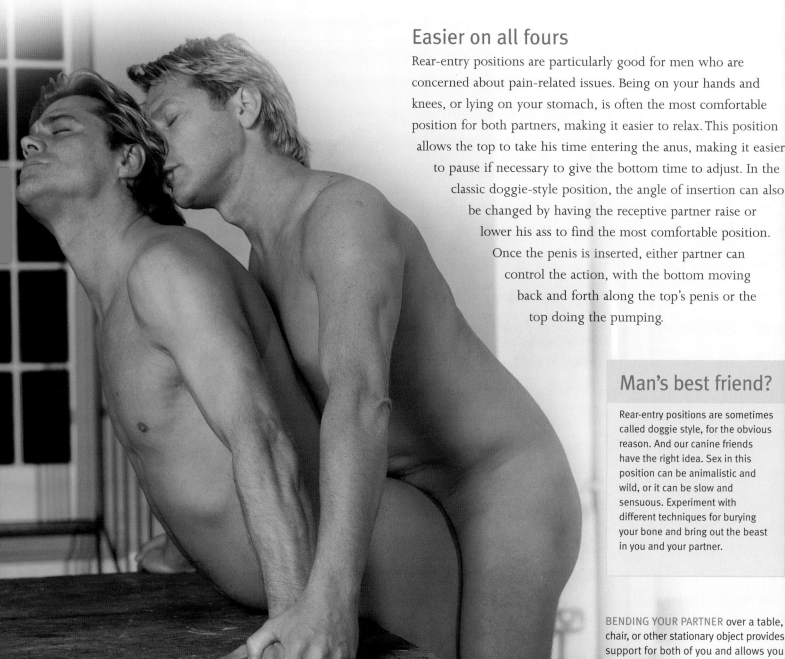

Man's best friend?

Rear-entry positions are sometimes called doggie style, for the obvious reason. And our canine friends have the right idea. Sex in this position can be animalistic and wild, or it can be slow and sensuous. Experiment with different techniques for burying your bone and bring out the beast in you and your partner.

BENDING YOUR PARTNER over a table, chair, or other stationary object provides support for both of you and allows you to thrust into him more deeply while staying in complete control.

VISUAL STIMULI ARE are often the
biggest turn-ons for us men, and
watching your penis enter your
partner can be very arousing.

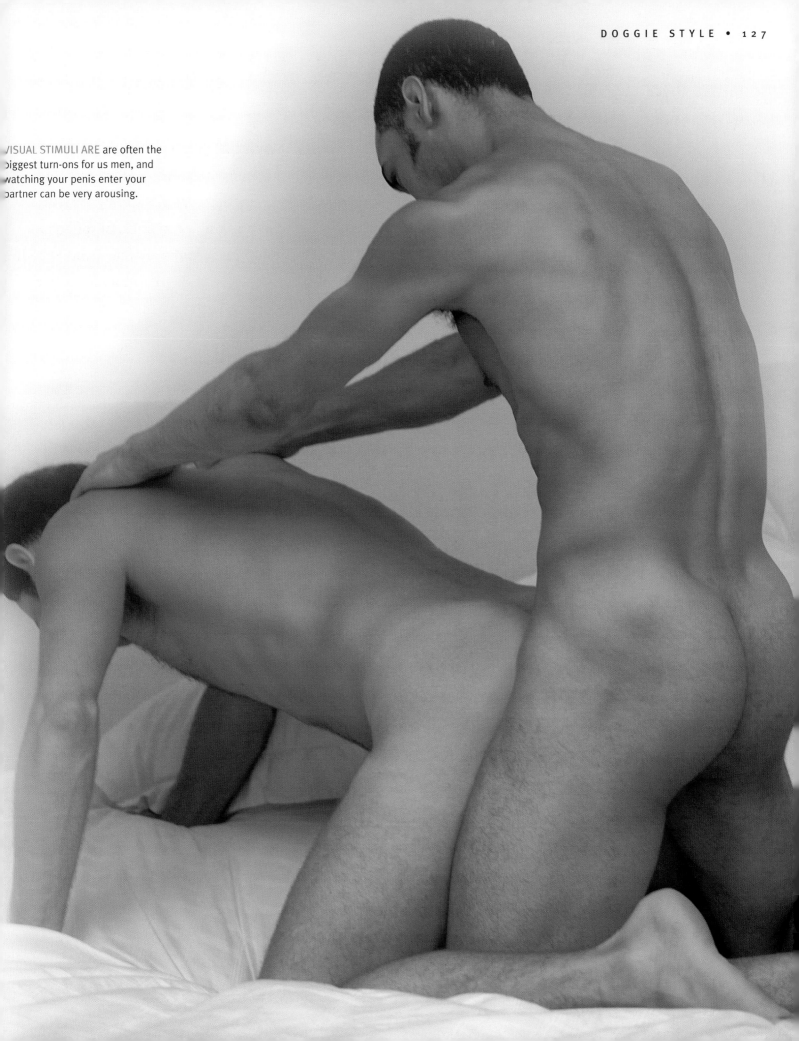

Standing position
Vertically challenging

The standing position is the sexual maneuver made famous in movie scenes where someone lifts his partner onto a desk or kitchen counter and they proceed to go at it. Standing sex tends to be associated with spontaneous, wild lovemaking because it reflects a passion and desire that have grown out of control. It may also be associated with having sex in unusual or confined places, where standing up is a necessity.

Standing to attention

Standing positions are actually variations on the missionary and doggie-style positions, the difference being that because the top is standing he can use the powerful muscles in his legs and thighs to achieve deeper, more powerful thrusting. The standing position can be done most effectively with the bottom positioned on the edge

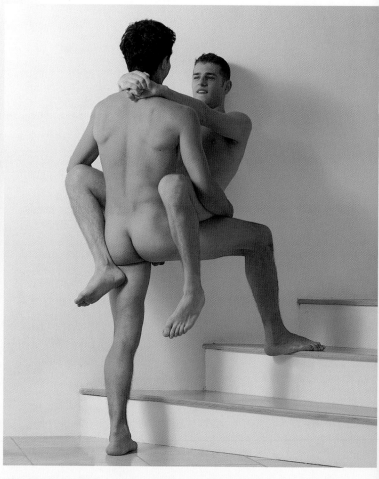

USING WALLS, STEPS, counters, and furniture for support makes standing sex a lot easier for both partners by removing arm strain.

THIS POSITION works best if the active (standing) partner is larger and/or stronger, because holding the body up places stress on the arms.

of a bed, counter, or other surface, and the top standing. This gives the top the most freedom of movement. It can also be achieved with the bottom's back against a wall, supported on the top's knee, or by his arms under the thighs. Penetration in this position may be limited, because of the difficulty of supporting a partner and thrusting at the same time, but it allows face-to-face contact and is a fun alternative to the standard missionary position.

A STANDING POSITION works best for partners of similar height. If you and your partner are of varying heights, you may find the angle of insertion uncomfortable.

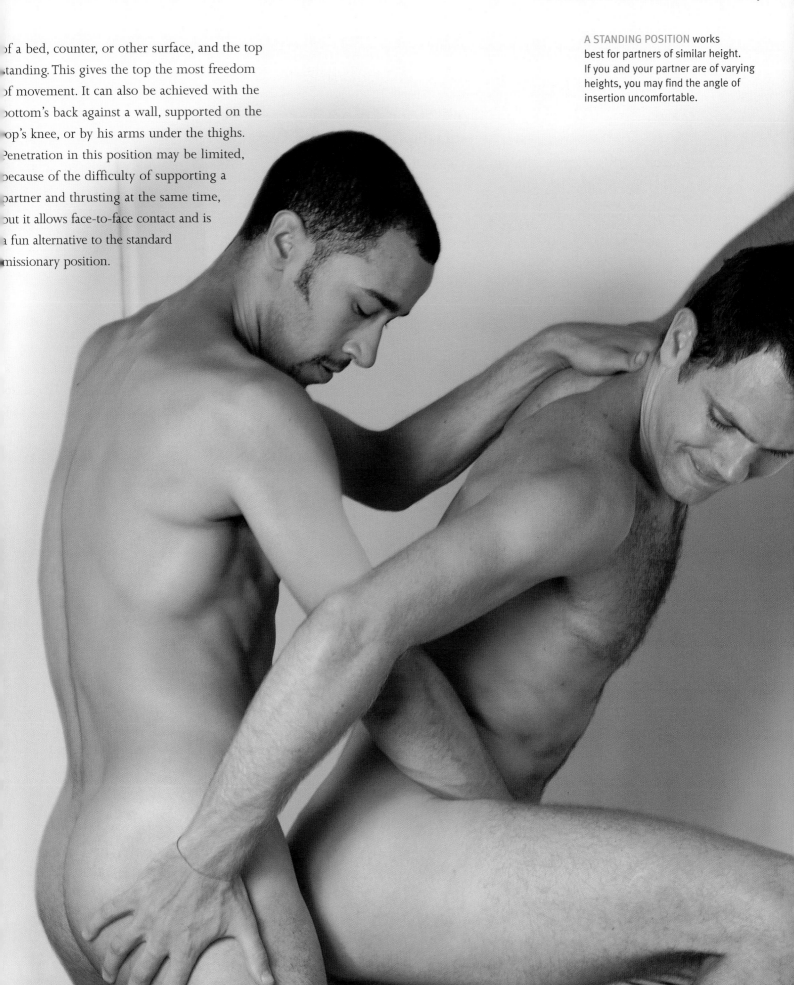

Turning position

One good turn deserves another

Who says you can't have the best of both worlds? With a little practice it's possible to switch from face-to-face sex to sex from behind (or vice versa) with barely a break in the action. It just requires moving a leg here and there. And why would you want to do this? I don't know, really, except that giving your partner a twirl on your stiffy might be fun. But actually it's because it lets you go at him from all different angles without starting and stopping, and this continuation feels really good. With no breaks in the action you're guaranteed not to miss a stroke.

Got your G spot?

What is considered the male G spot is actually the prostate, a walnut-sized gland that surrounds the urethra. The prostate's function is to make liquid to carry sperm. To find and stimulate it, insert a lubricated finger into the anus and press in the direction of the penis (toward the abdomen). Sustained stroking can be very pleasurable, and may induce orgasm.

One fluid movement

Obviously, this undertaking requires some patience and a few special rules. You can't just flip your partner over like a flapjack. You need to move carefully in order to make the transition as smooth as possible and not create too much of a break in the action. But, trust me, it can be done.

The biggest obstacle is legs, particularly getting them all where they need to be without getting tangled up. You can do this without taking your penis out of his ass, but you don't have to.

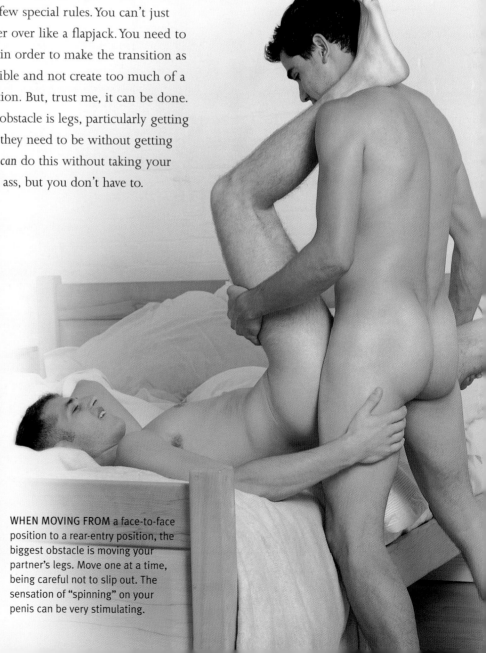

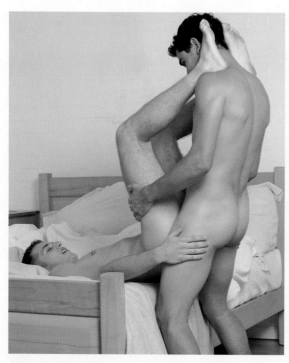

BEFORE ATTEMPTING ANY change in position, let your partner know what you're planning to do. Surprising him may cause him some discomfort.

WHEN MOVING FROM a face-to-face position to a rear-entry position, the biggest obstacle is moving your partner's legs. Move one at a time, being careful not to slip out. The sensation of "spinning" on your penis can be very stimulating.

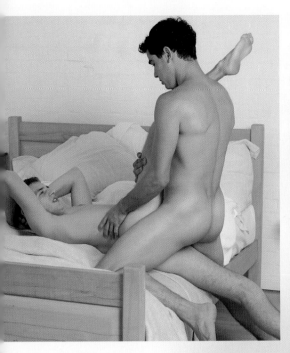

ONCE THE SECOND LEG is repositioned, the receptive partner can begin to turn onto his stomach. Help him by supporting his leg with your arm.

PUTTING ONE KNEE on the bed while sliding your partner's leg between your own will help to steady you while you reposition yourselves for more action.

WITH EVERYONE BACK in position, you're ready now to resume action from a new angle.

Removing your penis, having your partner turn over, and plunging it right back in can be incredibly hot. But if you want to do it while still staying inside, you can. In fact, you you can use each transitional move as an opportunity to do a little fucking from a different angle, which can be fun too.

One to another

The real point of moving from one position to the next is to create a series of different, yet similarly erotic sensations. Sometimes it's great to start out fucking with one position and end up climaxing with another, particularly if you and your partner like to come in different ways. Coming in his ass from behind and then turning him over so he can jack off while you pump him, for example, can be very arousing. Experiment to discover what feels best for both of you.

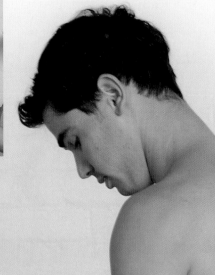

S&M

Domination, submission, and other sexual roles

S&M. These two letters conjure up all kinds of images: A man in leather spanking a guy over his knee; someone in a sling, his face hidden behind a mask as someone fucks him; a bare ass covered with the red welts left by a whip or a paddle. But S&M play is about much more than leather and rough sex. It is about the exchange of power between two (or more) people who are exploring the possibilities offered by assuming different sexual roles. It is about expanding personal boundaries, and discovering things about yourself by being vulnerable, both physically and emotionally.

An introduction to S&M

Although participating in various S&M activities can be a wonderful way to express your erotic personality, it isn't for everyone. The sex tends to be rougher, more elaborate, and potentially more emotionally demanding than typical, or vanilla, sex. But for those for whom S&M holds appeal, the possibilities are almost endless, and the rewards are potentially enormous.

In general terms, S&M involves interaction between a dominant partner and a submissive partner. But don't be fooled by these terms. Submissive does not necessarily mean weak-willed or passive, and dominant doesn't have to mean someone who controls every aspect of the sexual experience. In fact, they refer to who performs the action (the dominant partner) and who it is done to (the submissive partner). Although one person is doing the action and the other is having it done to him, both participants are contributing equally to the experience and both experience the rewards. One cannot have the experience without the other, and regardless of which position is taken, both partners have the ability to keep the action going or bring it to a halt.

What is S&M?

So what, exactly, is S&M, and how is it different from other sexual play? In broad terms, S&M centers on the taking and giving up of control.

For example, one partner may allow the other to bind his hands, blindfold him, spank him, put clamps on his nipples, or otherwise dominate him in the sense that he hands over the control of what happens to him and his body. S&M may or may not incorporate what we think of as typical sex acts (oral and anal sex, masturbation, ejaculation). More often than not it is less about

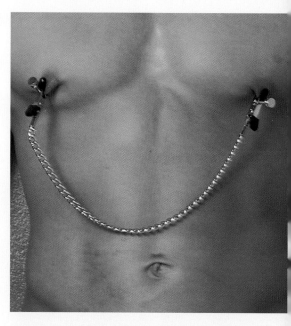

KNOWING HOW TO use the toys associated with S&M is crucial to keeping the play both erotic and safe. Nipple clamps are just one way of enhancing the experience.

THE CLOTHING ASSOCIATED with S&M is used to heighten the experience of playing different roles and assuming the characteristics of a different person, just as an actor's props help him "get into character."

Give me an "S"!

What's in a name? In the case of S&M, there are two founding fathers. The "S" stands for sadism, which is loosely defined as the act of deriving sexual gratification through inflicting pain or humiliation on others. The word comes from the name of the Marquis de Sade. An infamous figure in 19th-century France, the Marquis scandalized polite society with his outrageous public behavior and with the publication of books such as *Justine* and *120 Days of Sodom*, both of which portrayed a hedonistic world of sex and debauchery in which innocence is seen not as a virtue but as something to be destroyed. For his efforts the Marquis spent 27 years of his life in and out of jails and insane asylums, where he continued to write novels and plays.

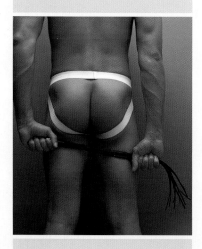

Give me an "M"!

Another writer, Leopold von Sacher-Masoch, gives us the "M"—or masochist—in S&M. The opposite of sadism, masochism is the deriving of sexual gratification from being humiliated, or from having pain inflicted on oneself. It is believed that Sacher-Masoch's sexual predilections stemmed from childhood incidents in which he was alternately showered with affection and then beaten by a female relative on whom he spied while she was with her lovers. Sacher-Masoch's feminine ideal—a strong, beautiful woman dressed in furs and wielding a whip—was immortalized in his classic erotic novel *Venus in Furs*.

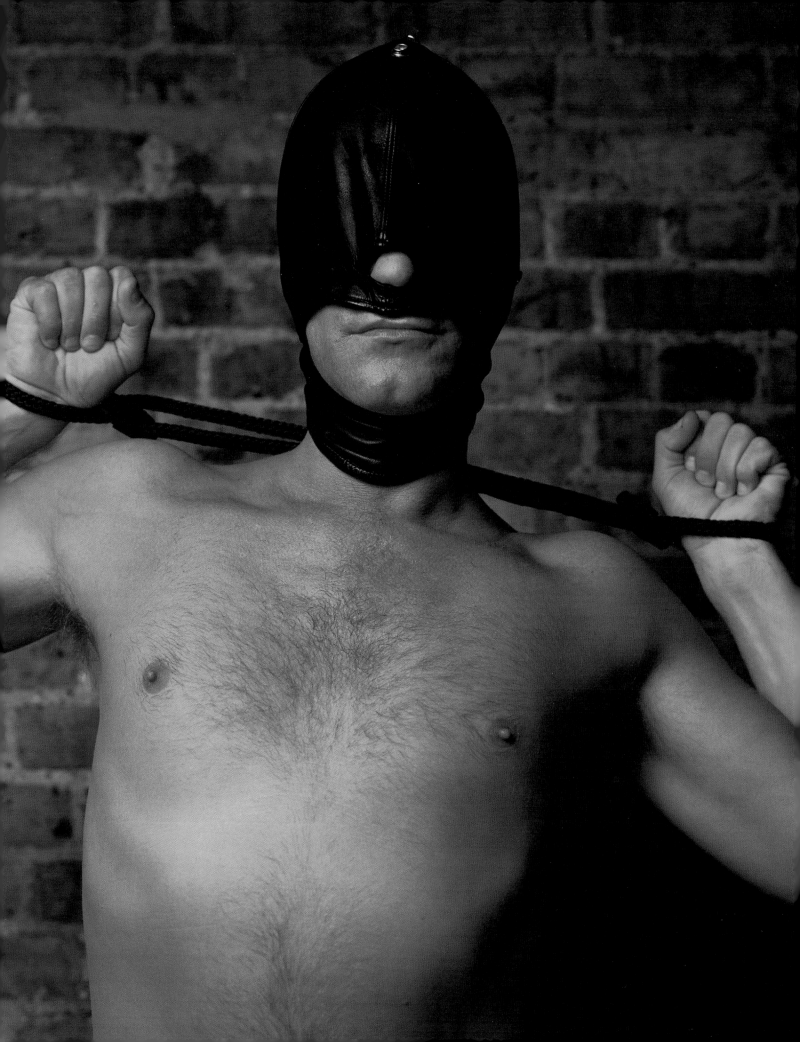

S&M tips

• When engaging in S&M play, be sure to establish a "safe word," which, when spoken by either participant, will end the play immediately in the event that it becomes too intense. Choose an unusual word, such as *rhinoceros* or *umbrella*, which is not likely to be spoken accidentally.

• If you decide to participate in S&M activities with someone you don't know well, be sure to establish your boundaries before you begin any activity. What's okay for you might not be okay for someone else.

• Use verbal communication to make a scene more interesting. Make the dialogue erotic and interesting rather than falling into bad porn-film talk.

• Experiment with alternating sensations to keep S&M play both erotic and exciting. Follow a hard spanking with a gentle massage, or the application of hot wax with an ice cube rubbed sensuously on the skin.

• If you use dildos during S&M play, be sure to cover them with a condom. Silicone can absorb body fluids, and it is possible to transmit infections and other sexually transmitted diseases through sharing sex toys.

• When using rope or other binding material in S&M activities, make sure you don't tie them too tightly and inadvertently cut off your partner's circulation.

• Don't attempt anything on a partner—such as body piercing, cutting, branding, or the use of hot wax or electric devices—that you aren't thoroughly familiar with.

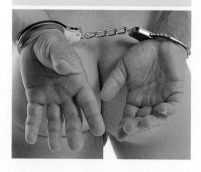

physical sexual release (coming) than about mental release and exploration. The S&M participant who enjoys being blindfolded and told to lick someone's boots, for example, may ultimately find it sexually arousing and come, but he may be even more aroused by the idea that he is doing something considered humiliating by others.

Costumes and equipment

As evidenced by the stereotypical image of an S&M participant being dressed in leather, S&M activities are often associated with various kinds of clothing such as leather vests, chaps, harnesses, and boots, as well as sexual aids such as handcuffs, whips, paddles, and butt plugs. As potentially erotic and exciting as these things are, they are really just props that aid participants in getting into the fantasy scenarios that lie at the heart of S&M play. A man who finds the idea of subjecting a partner to humiliation exciting, for example, may choose to dress himself as a police officer and act out the role of a cop forcing a "criminal" to suck his cock. Or a man who enjoys being "used" by other men for their sexual release may find extra excitement in wearing a mask to cover his face, rendering him even more anonymous to the men he allows to fuck him.

S&M play is a unique blend of fantasy and reality that allows you to become who you want to be, even if the role you choose is completely different from the role you play in real life. By acting out fantasies, S&M allows your sexual persona to emerge in a safe and liberating setting. A man who finds it difficult to give up control in his professional life, for example, may find it enormously satisfying to be tied up and ordered around by someone else during Alternatively, a man who is generally shy and soft-spoken in his everyday life can become a foul-talking, swaggering dominant when he puts on a leather jacket and sticks a cigar in his mouth. It's all about role reversal.

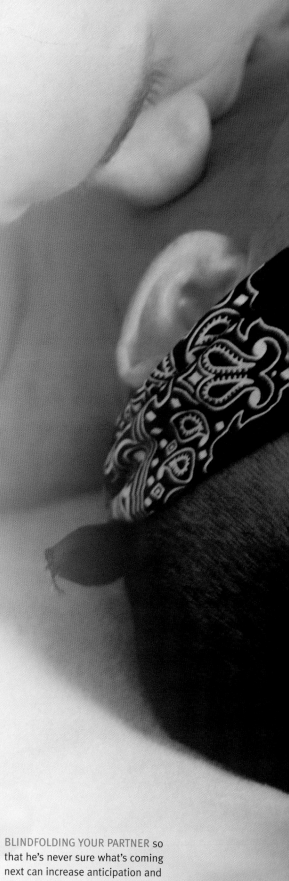

BLINDFOLDING YOUR PARTNER so that he's never sure what's coming next can increase anticipation and add excitement and mystery to your sexual play.

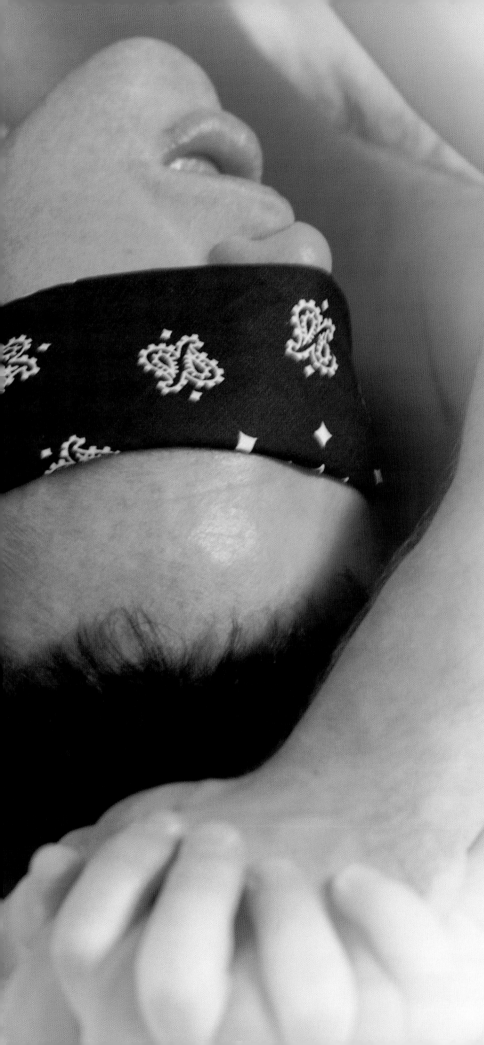

Keeping it non-extreme

You might think that S&M play isn't for you. But before you dismiss it as something only for other people, look more closely at the possibilities it provides. You don't have to dress up in leather and create elaborate scenarios to incorporate elements of S&M into your sexual life. Try tying your partner's hands behind his back with one of your neckties before you go down on him, or maybe let him blindfold you and describe a sexual fantasy in which he's a coach, burglar, or military officer using you for his sexual release. By exploring the many varied possibilities provided by S&M play, you might just surprise yourself by what you find arousing.

S&M as part of your lifestyle

If you find that you enjoy S&M and want to deepen your involvement in it, you will discover that there are numerous opportunities for doing so. The S&M community tends to be a very close one, and there are social organizations, bars, and sex clubs devoted to the lifestyle in most large cities. There are also some excellent internet resources and books for those interested in learning more about S&M (see pages 182–185 for more information).

The most difficult part of becoming involved in S&M is usually overcoming your fears and misunderstandings about it. By interacting with people in the S&M world you can find out more about who they are and what they do and see if it's something you want to partake in. And if you already know you're interested in exploring S&M, you'll find all kinds of opportunities for doing so.

As with any sexual activity, when considering partners for S&M activity keep your own mental and physical safety in mind. You know what you consider to be acceptable behavior, so stick to your guidelines and don't budge from them. It's that simple. S&M is about pushing your boundaries, but if someone makes you feel uncomfortable, or if you feel that you're being forced to do something, say no.

Toys
More than just playthings

Sex should be about playing, and what makes playing more fun than toys? Although we can get more than enough excitement from just using our bodies during sex, adding sex toys to our encounters can make things a little spicier. There's something for everyone in the toy chest, and finding out what you and your partners like to play with is an adventure in itself. Once you find your favorites, using them to enhance your sexual experiences—either alone or with a partner—becomes an excellent way to learn more about your sexuality, and to explore different ways of creating pleasure.

The tools of the trade

So what do we mean when we talk about sex toys? In the strictest sense, sex toys are devices of various types that are designed specifically for sexual use. These might include things like dildos, vibrators, butt plugs, nipple clamps, anal beads, or cock rings. But sex toys can also be things that weren't necessarily designed with sexual uses in mind. Handcuffs, for example, can be used in sexual play, as can objects such as feathers, clothespins, and really anything you can think of that can be used to stimulate yourself or a partner sexually.

The whole point of incorporating toys into your sex life is to add an element of fun and adventure. Many people are embarrassed about using sex toys because they think that it implies something is lacking in their life or in their relationships. This is a negative attitude based on a false assumption: that we should be happy with what we've got and not want anything else. Sex toys certainly *can* be used as alternatives for things that are missing from a relationship, but in general they're additions to our sexual lives, accessories that provide new elements of arousal to create a more positive, fun, and rewarding experience.

Let's take dildos, for example. Dildos are artificial penises made most often from rubber or silicone (although wooden, plastic, metal, and even glass versions are available). Dildos come in all shapes, sizes, and colors. Some people might look at a dildo and say that it's simply a substitute for a real penis, and in some ways they are right. But that's not what's important. What's important is how dildos can make your sex life more exciting.

Some men enjoy using dildos to stimulate themselves during masturbation, or perhaps during times when they don't have partners. Dildos can also be excellent learning tools for men who want to practice having anal sex or

IF YOU CREATE a sense of fun around using sex toys, it will remove any potential embarrassment, and allow you and your partner to enjoy the experience more.

Rubber up!

If you enjoy using sex toys—particularly dildos—with your partners, treat that faux phallus as if it's the real deal. Bodily fluids can stick to sex toys and, depending on what the toys are made of, be absorbed by them. If you share toys, you could also be sharing bacteria and viruses. Use rubbers, and change them before using the toys on the next guy.

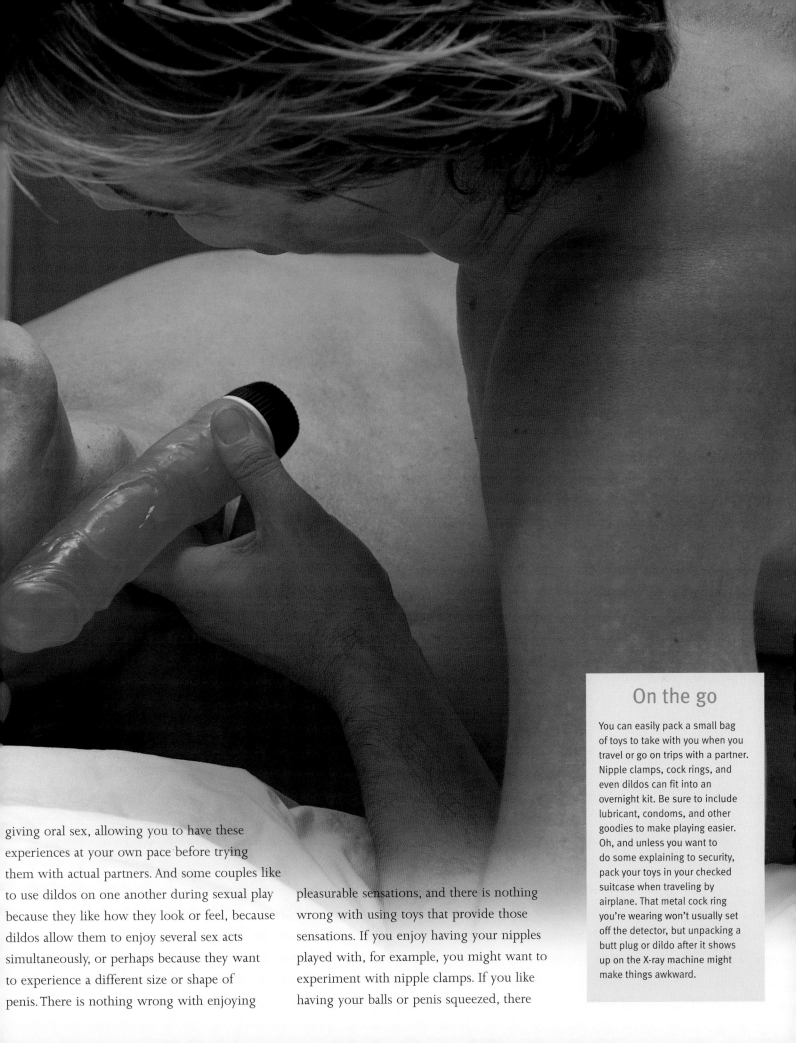

giving oral sex, allowing you to have these experiences at your own pace before trying them with actual partners. And some couples like to use dildos on one another during sexual play because they like how they look or feel, because dildos allow them to enjoy several sex acts simultaneously, or perhaps because they want to experience a different size or shape of penis. There is nothing wrong with enjoying

pleasurable sensations, and there is nothing wrong with using toys that provide those sensations. If you enjoy having your nipples played with, for example, you might want to experiment with nipple clamps. If you like having your balls or penis squeezed, there

On the go

You can easily pack a small bag of toys to take with you when you travel or go on trips with a partner. Nipple clamps, cock rings, and even dildos can fit into an overnight kit. Be sure to include lubricant, condoms, and other goodies to make playing easier. Oh, and unless you want to do some explaining to security, pack your toys in your checked suitcase when traveling by airplane. That metal cock ring you're wearing won't usually set off the detector, but unpacking a butt plug or dildo after it shows up on the X-ray machine might make things awkward.

are cock rings and straps available for such purposes. Try experimenting with butt plugs and anal beads that can be used to stimulate the rectum. There are even artificial mouths, rectums, and life-size dolls available for providing sexual gratification of various kinds.

The joy of toys

If you've never used sex toys as part of your sexual play then it's time to open your mind to the pleasurable possibilities they can bring. Start thinking about what kind of toys you might enjoy in your own sexual play. Think about what sensations you enjoy when it comes to sex, and about which body parts you enjoy having stimulated. Consider what you would do if you had toys to help you experience certain kinds of sensations or

SEX TOYS COME in an exciting range of shapes and colors, so rest assured that there are plenty of options to choose from. The samples, below, should give you a good idea of the kinds of toys that are available. Give one of them a whirl!

activities, or to help make the things you like doing even more enjoyable. Is this giving you some ideas? Good. Now let's talk about making it happen.

Once you've decided that playing with some toys might be fun (and it will be) you need to purchase them. Luckily, there are numerous options for buying sex toys. Many cities have entire stores devoted to them, with knowledgeable salespeople who will be happy to answer your questions. If you don't live in a city with a good sex-toy store, or if you prefer to be more discreet in your purchasing, there are also numerous catalogs and websites that offer sex toys for sale (see pages 182–185 for more information).

Don't be coy

As with using sex toys, the biggest obstacle to purchasing them can often be the embarrassment factor. It can be hard to ask the guy working behind a sex-store counter what a toy is and what it's used for. Looking at toys online or in catalogs can eliminate part of the problem, as can going shopping for toys with friends or with a partner. If you make a game out

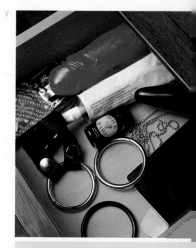

Toy box

Creating a special toy box to hold all of your sex toys is not only a practical way to store them, it can also be a lot of fun. Your chest can be as simple as a cardboard box or as elaborate as a trunk decorated in any way you like. Make a ritual out of opening your toy box when it's time to play; this will add to the sense of adventure. Keeping your chest well-stocked, and encouraging your partner to choose something new from it, can add an element of suspense and excitement to your sexual play.

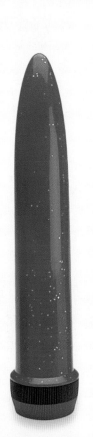

Basic vibrator

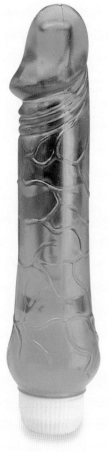

Penis-shaped vibrator

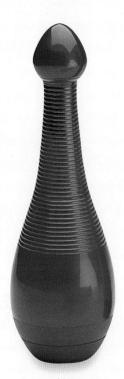

Textured butt plug

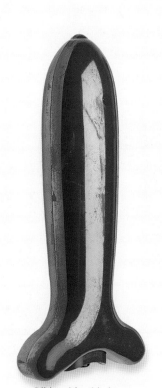

Dildo with wide base

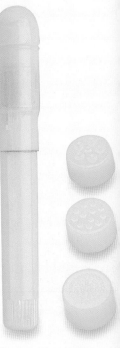

Vibrator with attachments

of it and approach looking for toys with an open, light-hearted attitude, you'll find that it's much less difficult than you imagine.

Slightly more difficult may be discussing the use of sex toys with a partner. You may find that your partner is very open to the idea, but it's possible that he'll have some reservations. In addition to feelings of embarrassment, your partner may feel that you want to use toys because something is missing from your relationship. It's important to assure him that this isn't the case, and that he understands that you want to try toys as a way of introducing a fresh spirit of adventure into your sex life.

Ease them in gently

As with any new sexual activity, don't just spring sex toys on a partner out of the blue. Talk about it beforehand. That way your partner can share any concerns he might have, and when it comes time to actually try out whatever toy you've chosen he'll be less stressed out about it. You might also want to start with something small (like a cock ring) and work your way up to more elaborate toys as your partner becomes more comfortable with them. If you make playing with and shopping for toys something you do together, then you'll retain that sense of fun that should

surround all kinds of sexual activity. Once your partner is comfortable with the idea of using sex toys, you can have a lot of fun looking for toys together or surprising each other with new goodies. Finding different ways to stimulate yourself or a partner will add excitement to your sex life and may even take it in new directions.

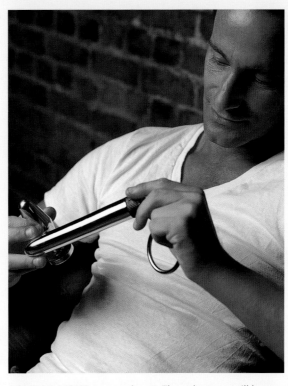

DON'T BE AFRAID to experiment. The only way you'll know whether you or your partner enjoy playing with toys such as butt plugs, vibrators, and cock rings is to try them out.

Dil-Do's and Don'ts

• Avoid using the same toys for anal and oral activities. Have separate ones for each.

• Dildos can absorb bacteria, so be sure to wash them after each use. Even better, use a condom on your dildo to prevent any risk of contamination.

• When sharing a dildo with a partner, put a condom on it and replace the condom before using the toy on your buddy.

• You can warm up dildos by placing them in warm (not hot) water for a few minutes before playing with them.

• Store dildos out of the sun and away from heat. Some dildos can leech color onto things they come into contact with, so be careful about what you wrap them in and put them next to.

• Always be sure to use water-based lubricants with sex toys, as oil-based ones can cause deterioration to the material.

• Bigger isn't always better. If you want to try the extra-large dildo or butt plug, work your way up to it.

• Get a dildo that has a wide base. It makes using it easier, and you don't want it to slide inside of you completely.

• For added fun, give your dildo a name. Telling your partner that he's going to get it from "Big Jake" or "Don Juan" tonight adds a sense of play to the experience.

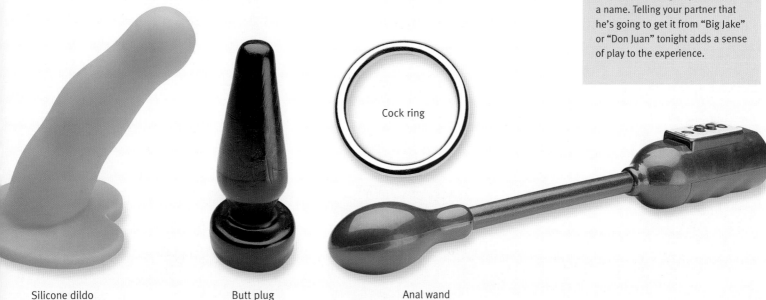

Silicone dildo   Butt plug   Cock ring   Anal wand

Exhibitionism

Standing tall and proud

When it comes to sex, do you like to show off? Does the idea of somebody watching arouse you? Many men enjoy the idea of someone watching them engaging in sexual play, either alone or with a partner. The thrill of exhibitionism comes from knowing that someone else is getting aroused by watching us get off. It puts us in a position of power; one in which what we do elicits sexual excitement in someone else and, in turn, ourselves. And by allowing someone to see us at our most intimate, we're breaking a taboo, even if that taboo exists only in our own minds.

An exhibition of yourself

In most cases, engaging in sexual activity in public or in public view is illegal. But exhibitionism can take many forms, and you don't have to put yourself in potentially risky situations in order to enjoy it. For example, having a partner watch while you masturbate or play with sex toys is one way of fulfilling the desire to be watched. So is engaging in play at a sex club with other people around, or in the privacy of your own home while a partner or someone else looks on.

The power of exhibitionism comes from putting on a show for others to watch. Therefore, in order to get maximum pleasure from the experience you should be good at performing. Gauge the effect your actions are having on your viewer or viewers, and act accordingly. Slow down or speed up the action to create dramatic tension. Don't think of having an orgasm as the main purpose, but as a pleasurable side benefit to the main event. The more you put into arousing your audience, the more you're going to be aroused yourself.

The fun and excitement of exhibitionism comes from having someone else watch us engage in sexual play. Not only does it make us feel as if we ourselves are sexually exciting, but there's the added turn-on of watching the other person become aroused as well. Exhibitionism is an exchange between the person showing off

and the person watching, and both players have important roles in the game. Without a doer and a watcher there can be no exhibitionism.

You can use exhibitionism to enhance sex with a partner in several ways. You can, for example, put on a sexy strip show for him. You can make the event as simple or as elaborate as you want to, incorporating music, costumes, props, and toys to create a fantasy scene you both enjoy. Similarly, you could stage a steamy photo session with your partner where you take turns recording one another stripping, masturbating, or engaging in acts you find arousing. The point is that you're showing off for your partner, arousing him and yourself by expressing your sexuality.

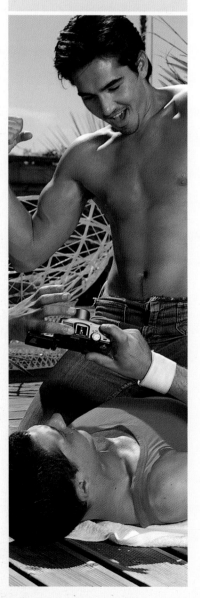

Show & tell

Exhibitionism doesn't have to be about revealing everything. It can be about giving hints as well. For example, wear a cock ring the next time you and your partner go out. At some point in the evening, slip his hand inside your pants just enough for him to feel the ring (or simply whisper in his ear that you're wearing one). Knowing it's there, and thinking about what you'll do when you get home, will get him all hot and bothered.

WHEN YOU FEEL good about your physique you bolster your self-esteem. Taking time to really look at yourself will help you get comfortable with your body, and teach you how to best show it off.

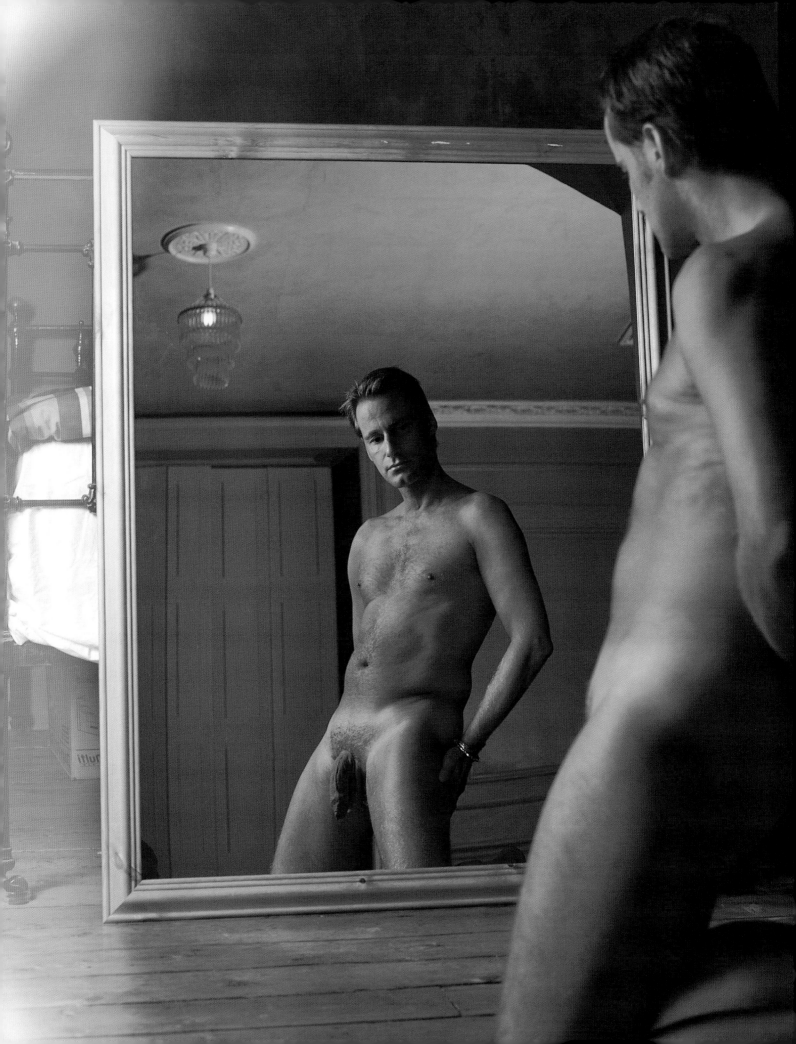

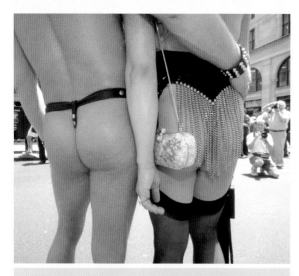

Peep show

In old-fashioned peep shows and burlesque routines, performers created sexual tension by gradually revealing different parts of themselves to their audiences. Often, they never even showed the whole thing. But still they drove their viewers wild. Why? Because they created an atmosphere of sensuality.

The power of exhibitionism comes from making someone wonder what else might be coming, from getting them to want more. By inciting the imagination, you incite the libido. How often have you seen a guy on the street and something about how he looked or acted made you imagine what might be underneath his clothes, or what he might be like in a sexual situation? That's the impression you want to give others when you show yourself off. And you can create it whether you're revealing everything or just a little bit.

Use the power of the imagination to increase the erotic draw when you show off for others. All kinds of clothes can be sexy, from the most conservative business suit to a revealing leather harness or jockstrap. Use what you wear (or don't wear) to make a statement about who you are as a person. Intrigue others by giving them hints to your sexual persona. Make them think about what you might have to offer and their interest in you will increase dramatically. Even walking around a beach or sex club totally naked, how you carry yourself can add another layer of erotic drama that will attract people to you for reasons other than what you look like without your clothes on.

Another exhibitionistic activity some men find very exciting is to create erotically charged situations in which they can show off for a partner. For example, if you're in the back yard and you know your partner can see you (but be sure the neighbors can't), you might want to strip down and let him watch you. Or you may want to go to your boyfriend's house one night and surprise him by putting on a little show outside his bedroom window (again, making sure you have privacy).

There are also places where exhibitionism is encouraged, at sex clubs, for example, or perhaps even on some nude beaches. If you find the idea of being watched by others exciting, take advantage of these places, either alone or with a partner. Use these experiences as ways to explore the power of your sexuality and to in turn be aroused by the reactions of others.

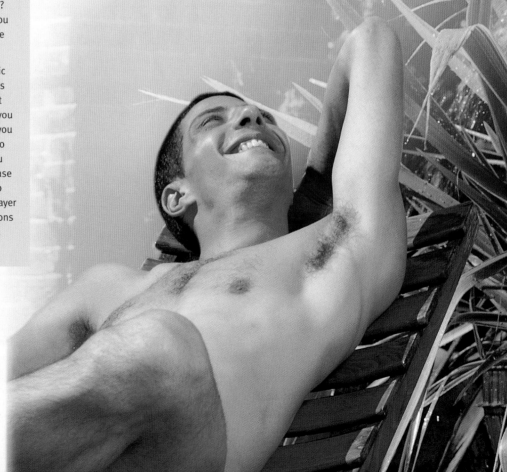

HAVING A PLAYFUL ATTITUDE about displaying your body will make showing off for a partner a fun experience.

Like what you see?

Very few of us are natural show-offs, especially when it comes to our bodies. But having confidence in yourself is the key to successful exhibitionism. You want anyone who's looking at you—whether it's a partner or someone seeing you for the first time—to be turned on. And this doesn't mean acting like a supermodel or the hottest guy on the beach; it means being comfortable with yourself. A man who is at ease with his body exudes natural charisma and is far sexier than someone who struts and poses.

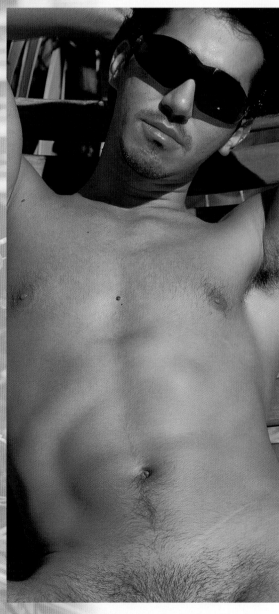

AN ATTRACTIVE GUY is a contented guy. By projecting an attitude of confidence about yourself, and feeling at ease about how you look, you will increase your overall appeal and draw other men to you.

Group sex

The more the merrier

Many men enjoy—or fantasize about—having sex with more than one person at a time. This may take the form of casual sex with a couple of buddies, sex with a larger group, or, most commonly, adding a third person (or being added) to an existing sexual relationship. Whatever the situation, the things you need to consider when engaging in sexual activity with more than one person at a time are pretty much the same. It calls for a little more planning but, when approached with the correct attitude, sex with more than one partner is something many men find very rewarding.

Safety in numbers?

The reasons for having sex with more than one partner at a time vary from man to man. Some men simply like the variety offered by different types of guys, while others enjoy watching a couple having sex or being watched themselves. Some partnered men find that adding a third person to the mix introduces a spark of excitement into a relationship, and some men get a thrill out of being added to someone else's relationship. As with any sexual activity, you can't predict who will be aroused by group sex or why. This intriguing factor makes group sex all the more taboo and mysterious.

There is one unbreakable rule about three-ways and group sex, though: if you don't enjoy it, don't pressure yourself or anyone else into doing it. For many of us, sex with more than one partner can trigger a lot of emotional responses that can be difficult to deal with. Even when the idea of sex with multiple partners sounds thrilling,

Easy as 1, 2, 3

If you and your partner are thinking of having a three-way, following a few simple rules will go a long way in preventing misunderstandings.

1 Discuss your reasons for wanting to try a three-way. If you aren't in agreement on the purpose of it, or if one of you feels pressured to try it, don't do it.

2 Set the ground rules *before* you play. If there are certain activities that are off limits or reserved for you and your partner (kissing and anal sex, for example), make it clear right up front.

3 Agree that it's okay for either of you to stop the action at any point if you begin to feel uncomfortable, frightened, jealous, or sad. Sometimes unexpected emotions arise once the action starts.

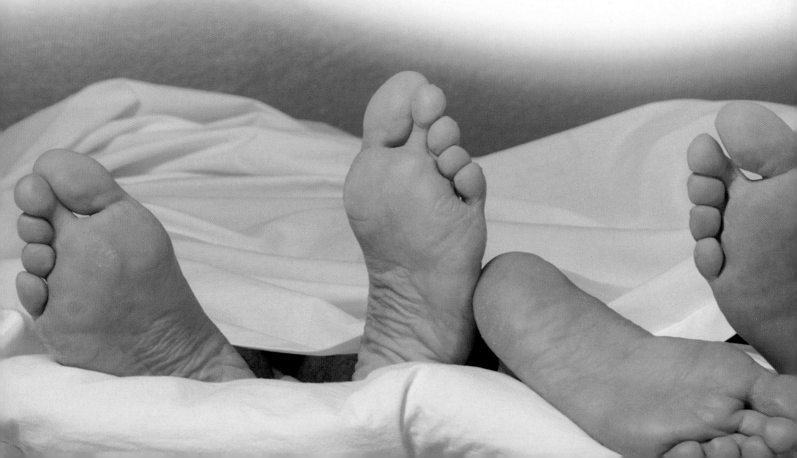

DOUBLE THE PARTNERS can mean twice the pleasure, but it also means paying attention to the needs and emotions of another person.

ometimes the reality is a different story. So if
ou know you won't be able to handle the added
motional pressures associated with group sex, or
f you try it and find you don't enjoy it, remember
hat you don't have to do it.

More than skin deep

Now that that's out of the way, let's talk
about what makes sex with more than one
guy both unique and challenging. I think
it's pretty obvious: with more than one
other person involved there are more than two
sets of emotions involved. Sure, the logistics
of dealing with an added penis, another set of
hands, and one more mouth to do something
with are tricky, too, but really it's about dealing
with feelings and personalities, not just bodies.
The dynamics of a multiple-partner situation
are more complicated than they are with just
two people. It's easy for someone, intentionally
or not, to feel left out, jealous, or unhappy,
and maintaining sexual excitement and
emotional satisfaction for everyone
involved can be a difficult balancing act.

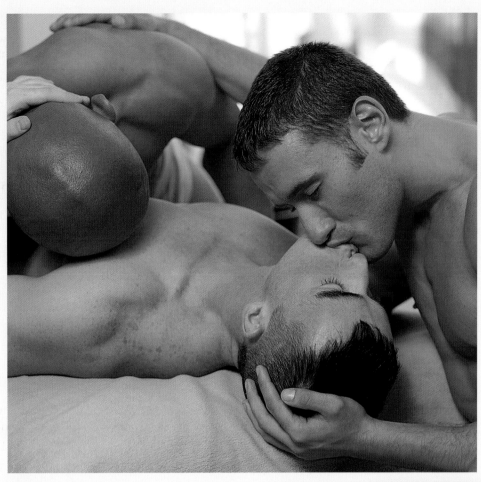

ADDING SOMEONE ELSE to your relationship can give both of you opportunities to play with different
roles and experiment with new, erotic positions.

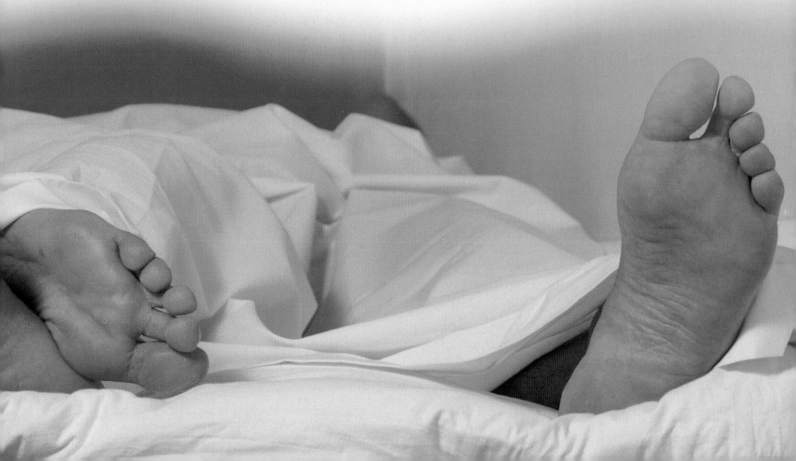

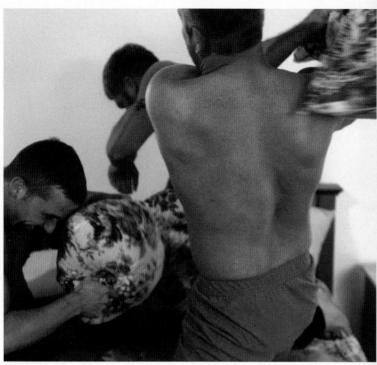

PLAYFULNESS BETWEEN PARTNERS can help ease tensions and encourage light-hearted contact in preparation for sexual activity.

Obviously, a three-way or orgy with anonymous partners at a sex club or with fuck buddies in a casual setting is generally about simply getting off, in which case your concerns are mostly about making sure you play safely. Since three-ways involving partners are the most common form of group sex, and have the greatest potential for problems, we'll focus on them.

You, me, and him

Whether you are adding a third guy to your existing relationship or you are being added as the third guy to another partnership, the key to making group sexual experiences work is to create sexual energy that encompasses all three partners. What this means in practical terms is making sure that each partner is receiving attention and is being included in the action.

It's very common in three-ways for two of the partners to be more attracted to each other than they are to the third person. This is especially true for couples who find different types of men attractive, and who incorporate a third man into their sex lives who appeals to one of them more

than the other. What happens, of course, is that the two guys who are really into each other spend more time with one another, leaving the third guy out. If this happens—and you're not the odd man out—then at least have the decency not to heap praise on the cute one you like in front of the guy who's feeling neglected.

As with all sex, the easiest way to make sure each participant gets what he wants from a group sex experience

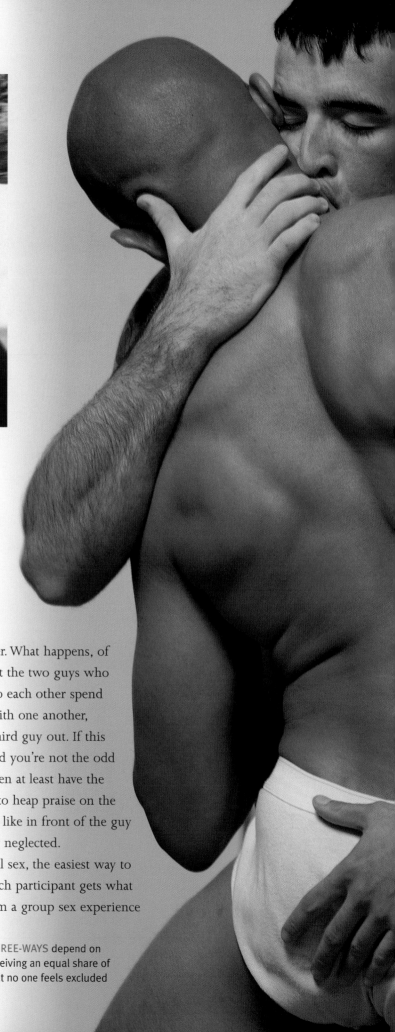

SUCCESSFUL THREE-WAYS depend on each partner receiving an equal share of attention, so that no one feels excluded or in the way.

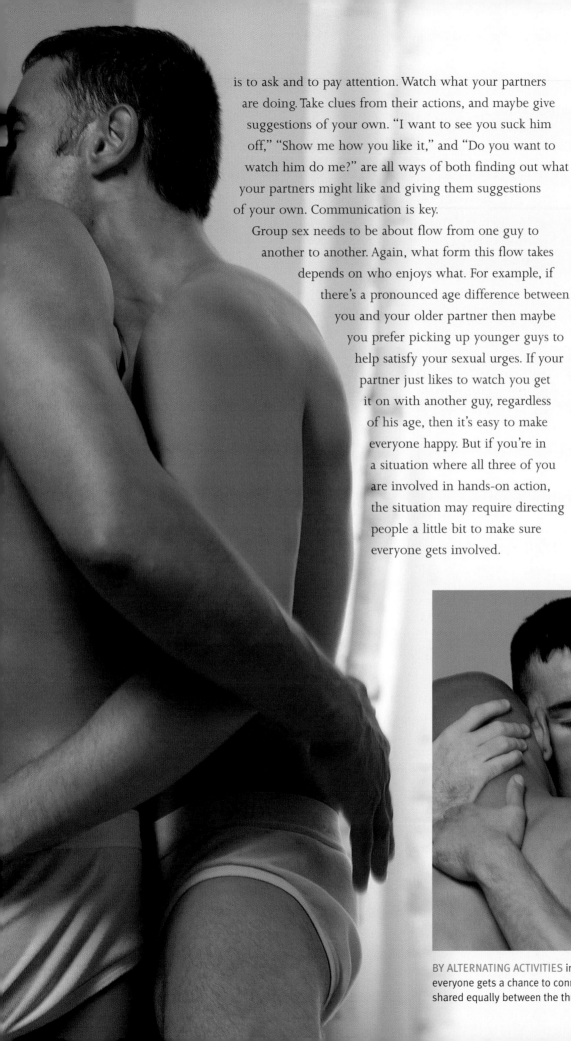

is to ask and to pay attention. Watch what your partners are doing. Take clues from their actions, and maybe give suggestions of your own. "I want to see you suck him off," "Show me how you like it," and "Do you want to watch him do me?" are all ways of both finding out what your partners might like and giving them suggestions of your own. Communication is key.

Group sex needs to be about flow from one guy to another to another. Again, what form this flow takes depends on who enjoys what. For example, if there's a pronounced age difference between you and your older partner then maybe you prefer picking up younger guys to help satisfy your sexual urges. If your partner just likes to watch you get it on with another guy, regardless of his age, then it's easy to make everyone happy. But if you're in a situation where all three of you are involved in hands-on action, the situation may require directing people a little bit to make sure everyone gets involved.

Group gropes

Establishing a network of buddies for regular group play can be a fun way to create a comfortable, safe environment for participants to explore multi-partner sexual activity. For example, putting together a group of guys who meet up for JO sessions, oral sex, erotic massage, or other types of play provides you and your friends with opportunities to express yourselves sexually, while also removing some of the fears that often accompany such activities.

Similarly, many cities have sex clubs—public and private—where you can experience having sex with multiple partners. These places, too, can provide good opportunities for trying out three-ways or group action, either on your own or with a partner. If you're interested in visiting a sex club, take a little time to investigate. Perhaps S&M is your thing, in which case you have only to do a little homework to find the club that's right for you.

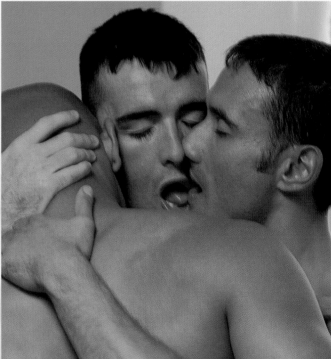

BY ALTERNATING ACTIVITIES in a three-way between your partners, everyone gets a chance to connect with each other, and roles are shared equally between the three of you.

Fetishes

Whatever turns you on

Do you get excited when you think about a man in a military uniform, or when you see a guy wearing a business suit? Does the smell of leather get you fantasizing about engaging in certain sexual activities? For many of us there are particular things that, for whatever reason, stir our erotic desires. Maybe they remind us of a great sexual encounter we've had, or perhaps we associate them with a sexual fantasy we've yet to fulfill. Are there specific things—clothing, body types, objects—that get you all worked up? If so, these things may be fetishes for you.

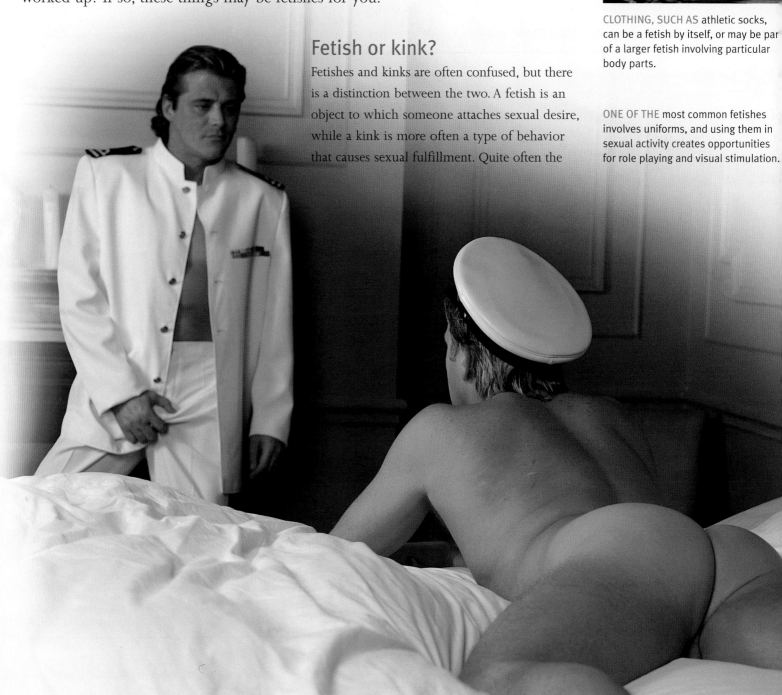

CLOTHING, SUCH AS athletic socks, can be a fetish by itself, or may be part of a larger fetish involving particular body parts.

ONE OF THE most common fetishes involves uniforms, and using them in sexual activity creates opportunities for role playing and visual stimulation.

Fetish or kink?

Fetishes and kinks are often confused, but there is a distinction between the two. A fetish is an object to which someone attaches sexual desire, while a kink is more often a type of behavior that causes sexual fulfillment. Quite often the wo are closely linked. The truest definition of a fetish is an object, such as a charm, statue, or totem, which is believed to have magical properties. A fetish is often worshipped or adored because it is thought to protect those who adore it. Sexually, a fetish is an object, or often a body part, with which a person associates sexual pleasure. For example, some men find feet to be very sexually exciting. Touching feet, massaging them, or even just looking at them can bring some guys to orgasm. A foot fetishist may enjoy licking feet, having a partner rub his feet on his face or body, or simply seeing pictures of feet.

Inanimate objects can also be the focus of a fetish. Leather, for example, is a very common fetish. Many men enjoy the smell, taste, and feel of leather. They enjoy wearing it or looking at other men wearing it. For someone with a leather fetish, items made out of the material, such as boots, may become objects of intense desire. Licking someone's boots, seeing a man in a leather harness, or being spanked with a leather belt can be an incredible turn-on.

You name it

Pretty much anything can become a fetish, from common items such as socks, jockstraps, or boxer briefs, to more unusual items. While writing my sex advice columns I heard from men who were turned on sexually by things as diverse as G.I. Joe action figures, particular brands of athletic shorts from the 1970s, and even certain TV shows. For them, these items were terribly arousing, and they used them in various ways to achieve sexual fulfillment, sometimes by wearing them during sex or by using them as part of masturbatory activity.

Where do these fetishes originate from? Fetishes develop because we have certain associations with the object at the center of the fetish. Many men, for instance, find uniforms incredibly sexually exciting. Military, police officer, fireman, and athletic clothing can be sexually arousing because maybe we like how

men who wear such clothes look, or because we find the characteristics of men who wear these uniforms, as part of their work, appealing.

There are many different reasons for the development of fetishes. Sometimes they're rooted in childhood, a time when we're developing sexually, and sights, sounds, smells, and tastes often take on a larger-than-life meaning. Often they develop out of our sexual fantasies. And sometimes they're a result of particularly fulfilling sexual encounters that we then associate with a particular object.

Anything to anyone

We tend to think of fetishes as something unusual, but anything can be a fetish, including body types. You might really get off on balding men, or men with hairy chests or big noses. Or maybe you're particularly attracted to men who are Irish, Japanese, or Mexican. Skin and hair color, accents, and other distinguishing characteristics can all be fetishes if you attach specific sexual desires to them.

Remember when

Many fetishes are related to particular times in our lives when we experienced strong sexual feelings. Think back to your teenage years. If you were on a sports team in school, for example, and you fantasized about (or actually experienced) getting it on with one of the other players in the locker room, then you might have a lingering erotic attraction to sports uniforms or paraphernalia. Or perhaps you used to masturbate while smelling someone's worn underwear or sweaty T-shirt? This is a sense-specific fetish—it's the odor that turns you on. These kinds of musky smells may continue to arouse you and rekindle the memories long after the original incident is over, or the object of your attraction has disappeared from your life. The fetish, however, allows you to relive the experience all over again.

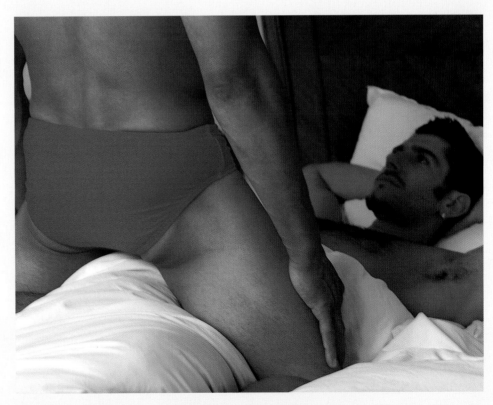

A FETISH FOR athletes or for athletic clothing provides numerous opportunities for acting out sexual fantasies. Experimenting with different scenarios can be incredibly exciting.

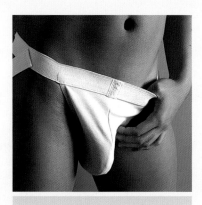

Make it brief

Underwear and jockstraps are a very common fetish, and one of the easiest to have fun with. The smell, look, and feel of them can all be powerful turn-ons. If you have an underwear fetish, explore it by collecting different types of garments and seeing which ones appeal to you the most.

A fetish in itself is not harmful. Associating sexual desire with objects, body parts, or even types of people is not a negative thing. In fact, fetishes can be fun to play with sexually, and can form the core of very satisfying sexual fantasies and encounters. Having a lover dress up in leather or in a particular kind of clothing, for example, can be extremely rewarding, and being particularly attracted to certain types of guys is not necessarily unhealthy.

More than a fetish

A fetish becomes a problem when it interferes with experiencing a wider range of sexual satisfaction and when it becomes a replacement for interpersonal experiences. If the only way you can become aroused is by having your partners dress up like clowns, for example, you're creating a behavioral pattern that

doesn't allow for other ways of achieving sexual pleasure. If you limit your sexual fantasies or real-life encounters solely to licking men's shoes or masturbating with used jockstraps, then there's probably something holding you back from relating to the men who wear these items in other ways. You need to broaden your sexual horizons.

It's not all or nothing

A fetish should not become the center of your sex life. Getting hot over certain types of underwear is fine, but only being able to make love to men wearing them isn't. Getting hard when you see a tall, dark-haired, handsome Italian man also isn't a problem, but being obsessed with finding an Italian lover to the point of excluding all other men from possible consideration is limiting yourself because of an obsessive fantasy.

Found your fetish?

The beauty of a fetish is that often for every fetish you have there's someone out there who gets off on you having it. For instance, if you're into licking boots or shoes, there are lots of guys out there who are into you licking theirs. If worshipping a hairy-chested man is your thing, there are plenty of hairy-chested men whose thing is being worshipped by you. So how do you go about finding one another? Bars and clubs centered on certain activities are always the best places to start. Many bars now hold fetish nights where specific items of clothing (leather or underwear, for instance) are the sole focus of the evening. Internet sites and personal ads are other excellent ways to find guys who appreciate your fetish.

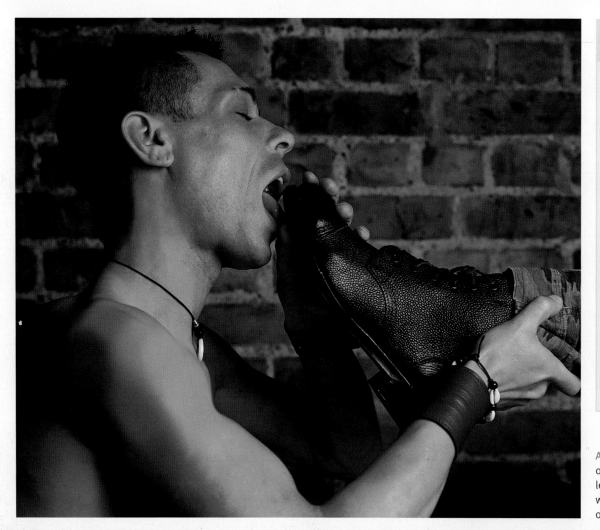

A SHOE OR BOOT fetish may be based on enjoying the smell or taste of leather, but it can also be associated with intensely pleasurable memories of a certain person or experience.

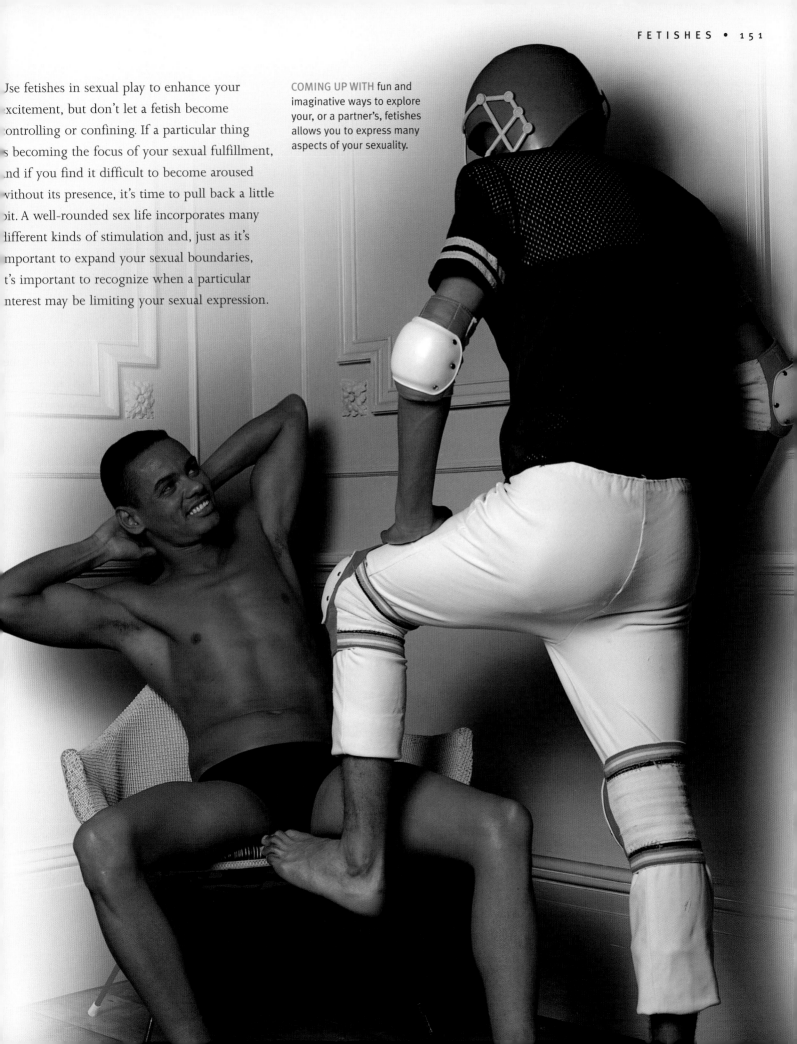

Use fetishes in sexual play to enhance your excitement, but don't let a fetish become controlling or confining. If a particular thing is becoming the focus of your sexual fulfillment, and if you find it difficult to become aroused without its presence, it's time to pull back a little bit. A well-rounded sex life incorporates many different kinds of stimulation and, just as it's important to expand your sexual boundaries, it's important to recognize when a particular interest may be limiting your sexual expression.

COMING UP WITH fun and imaginative ways to explore your, or a partner's, fetishes allows you to express many aspects of your sexuality.

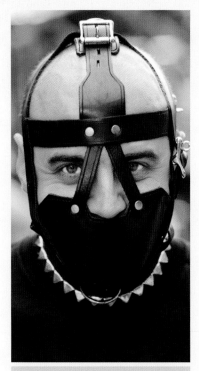

Kinks

You really got me going

What's kinky? Wearing a latex body suit? Being tied up and having hot wax dripped on you? Letting someone put on rubber gloves and slide his grease-covered fist inside your ass? Your notion of what's kinky may be vastly different from mine, or from that of the guy who's standing in the corner of the bar and who you're thinking about taking home later for a little fun. When it comes to kinks, it's all based on personal perspective, personal experience, and personal sexual boundaries. But one thing that all kinks have in common is that they express our sexual desires in unique ways.

Behind the mask

Because kinks are often associated with certain kinds of clothing, accessories, and behaviors, many people automatically equate them with S&M. Although S&M certainly can be a kink, not all kink-related activities involving S&M gear are about S&M.

Does this sound complicated? It's really not. It's just the difference between a costume and the role that's being played by the person who's wearing that costume.

Take our friend in the photograph above, for example. Maybe he is into S&M. But perhaps he just likes wearing the mask and collar. Perhaps for him the turn-on is having his mouth covered so that he has to rely on other ways of communicating with his partners. It may be that his sexual play involves elements of S&M, but it doesn't necessarily have to.

Too often we get caught up in what our interests and desires mean, but this is missing the point. Really, the only thing that's important is that we enjoy both what interests us and what we desire. Just because you favor an element of a particular kink or fetish doesn't mean you have to commit to it completely.

Setting kinks straight

Kinks and fetishes are often strongly connected in people's minds. In fact, a kink is more about enjoying a type of behavior or a type of activity, while a fetish is an object that may be related to the activity. A leather fetish, for example, can form the basis for an interest in S&M, or a fetish for latex and rubber may grow into an involvement with dressing up in clothes made from these materials.

Like fetishes, sexual kinks have also gotten something of a bad reputation. We tend to think of "kinky" sex as being something really unusual or something that only a handful of people participate in. In reality, what used to be considered kinky sex is sometimes now very common. S&M, for instance, isn't considered as kinky as it once was, thanks primarily to wider discussions of its appeal and its usefulness in sexual play. Like anything else that is adopted by a wider audience, sexual activities that were once seen as slightly perverse suddenly cease to be out of the ordinary.

Not extreme, just different

A kink is an interest in a particular type of sexual play that doesn't fall neatly into any of the more commonly discussed types of sex. Pain can be one. So can dressing up. Role play is another good example of a sexual kink. Of course, all these activities can be incorporated into more conventional types of sex play, so in and of themselves they aren't really kinky. It's more how they're done that lifts them above the commonplace and makes them something different. Rather than seeing kinks as extremes, they should be viewed as different forms of more basic sexual activities.

A lot of guys enjoy a little bit of nipple pinching, biting, or spanking in their sex play. But some men like to take it further, perhaps by incorporating piercing, cutting, or even branding into their sex lives. For them the pain itself is a fetish, but the infliction of pain or having pain inflicted on themselves on a grander scale becomes the behavioral kink. A common behavior that is magnified and intensely focused makes something a kink.

Again, it's about what we *do* that defines a kink. Many of us find various types of clothing sexy, and may use them in our sexual activities. But someone, for whom dressing up is a kink, may go way beyond that, creating elaborate scenarios that involve costumes and props. A rubber fetishist, for example, might encase his whole body in rubber, and use being bound in rubber as a focus for his sexual play.

FOR MEN WHO find certain textures (such as latex or rubber) erotic, wearing or seeing someone wearing items made from that material is a real turn-on.

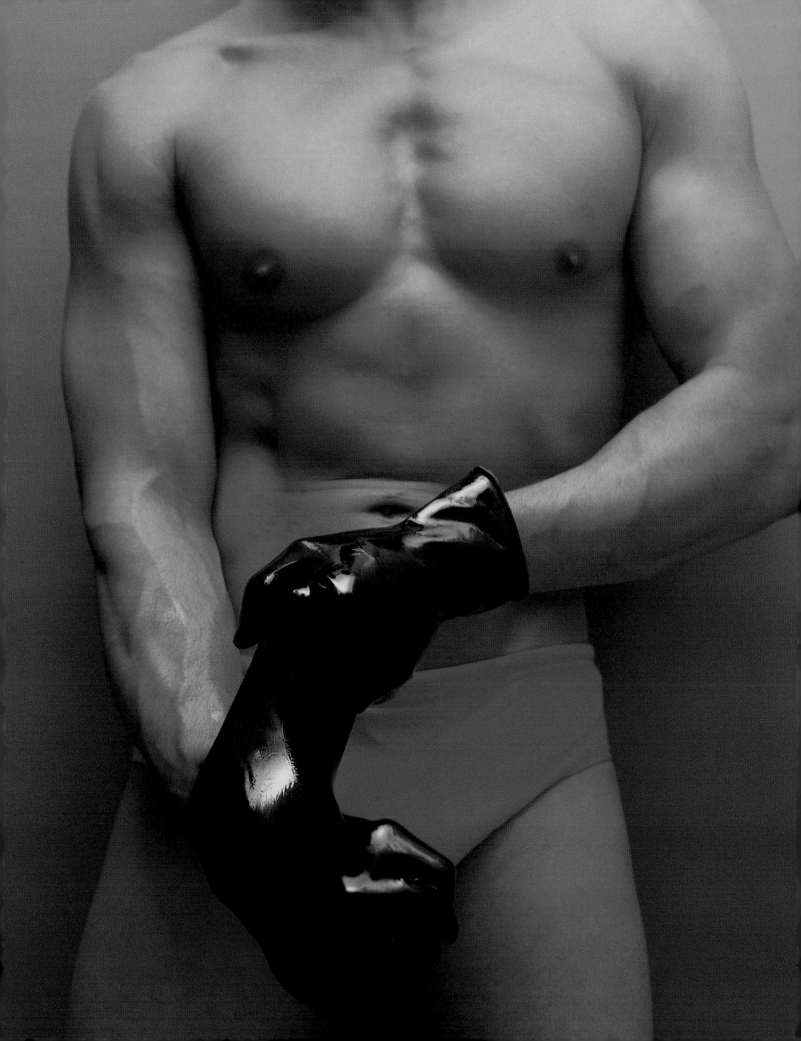

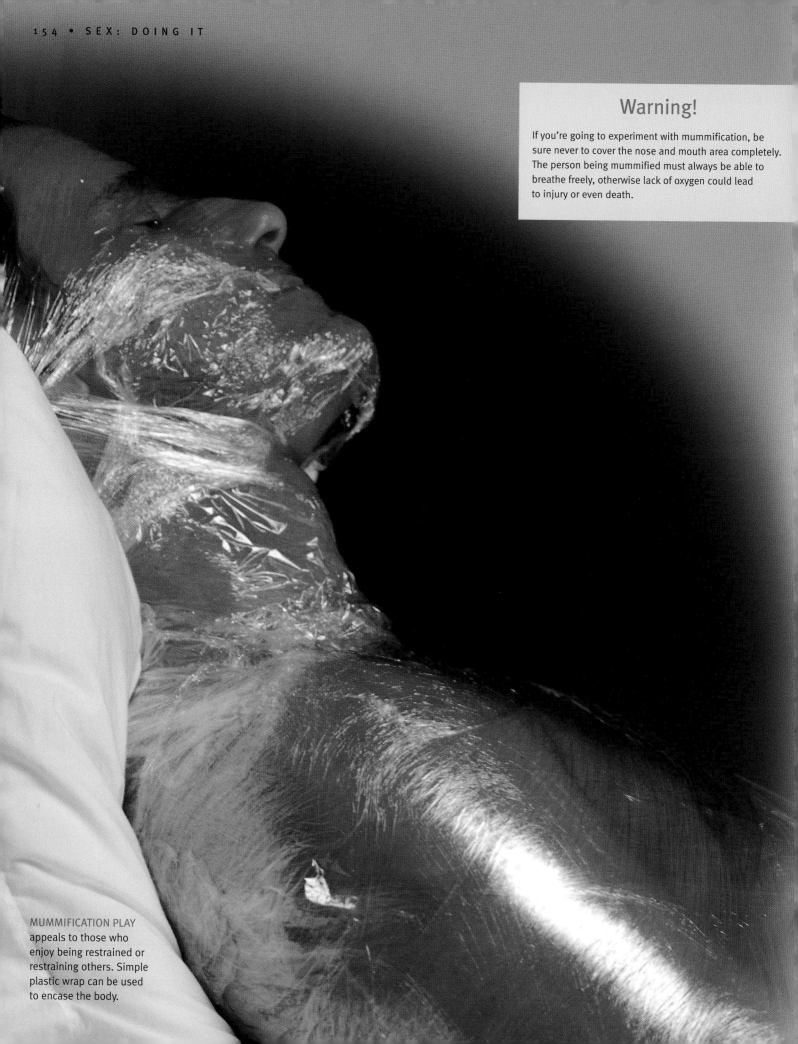

Warning!

If you're going to experiment with mummification, be sure never to cover the nose and mouth area completely. The person being mummified must always be able to breathe freely, otherwise lack of oxygen could lead to injury or even death.

MUMMIFICATION PLAY appeals to those who enjoy being restrained or restraining others. Simple plastic wrap can be used to encase the body.

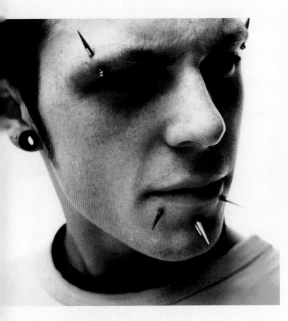

Someone with an interest in role play may take that interest to the next level, engaging in infantilism maybe, where an adult dresses and acts like an infant while a partner cares for him.

Why the bad press?

As odd as they can sometimes appear, kinks aren't bad things, and it's unfortunate that the very words "kink" and "kinky" imply some level of disrespectability. Dressing up like and pretending to be a horse might not be your thing, but there are people who actually love it. (Really. It's called pony play.) The thought of engaging in urine play (known as golden showers) or in fisting, where a partner's whole hand is inserted into the rectum, might make you cringe, but some guys find it their idea of heaven. As with any sexual activity, kinks might not be for you, but that doesn't mean they shouldn't be for someone else.

It's important to remember that a kink is only emotionally and physically "healthy" when it doesn't involve behavior that exploits someone else or results in emotional or physical harm to a partner. Sexual activity can contain elements of pain, dominance and submission, bondage, and other potentially "harmful" practices and still be positive experiences for everyone involved, but only when such activity is consensual.

MANY PEOPLE EXPRESS their kinks in physical ways, such as by piercing their bodies or getting tattoos that reflect their personalities or interests.

Exploring your personal kinks might not be as easy as participating in other forms of sexual play, but there are definitely options. In some instances, clubs and organizations have formed around certain types of sexual interests (dressing up and role playing, for example). These provide excellent outlets for expressing your interests and for learning more about the options available to you.

Introducing partners to your kinks is also an option open for you. Your lover might not ultimately be into having you wrap him up in plastic wrap (a practice called mummification) or in piercing your skin with dozens of pins, but you never know. Your interest may become something you can share.

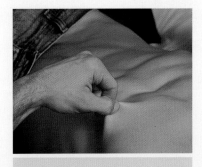

Just a pinch

Whether something is kinky or not depends entirely on your perspective. A completely ordinary, run-of-the-mill activity for you may really push someone else's sexual boundaries. Much more important than giving our particular sexual behaviors a label, however, is understanding why we enjoy them. When we know why a kink appeals to us, we learn a great deal about ourselves and our desires.

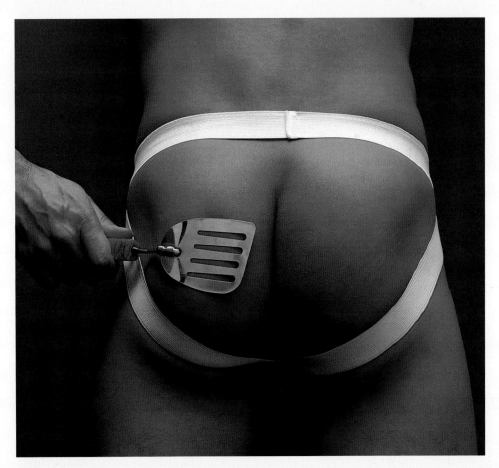

COMMON HOUSEHOLD ITEMS can often be put to new kinky uses. All it takes to get your imagination going is a playful attitude—and a little resourcefulness.

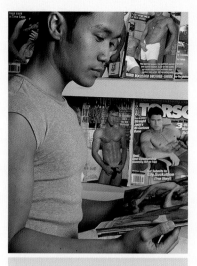

Pornography
A means of arousal

The word *pornography* was coined from the French for "writing about prostitutes." From this inauspicious beginning, porn has evolved to encompass writing, photography, film, art, and even computer-based media that explore sex in all its forms. Once considered something to buy in seedy stores and hide beneath mattresses, erotic materials are now sold and enjoyed openly. Whereas once the use of porn was more or less confined to getting off alone while looking at pictures of naked people, now it is often used as a way to encourage and heighten sexual activity between partners.

Porn-O-Rama

So how can you use porn to make your sex life more exciting? Try one of the following suggestions. Use them as starting points for coming up with your own ideas. And be creative. The more you put into the activity, the more you'll get out of it.

1 Ask your lover to rent or buy a porn video that he finds exciting and watch it together. Talking about what you find arousing in the video may inspire some cinematic fireworks of your own.

2 Pick up a collection of erotic fiction. Get naked and read a story to your partner while he masturbates for you.

3 Make your own porn video by taping yourself getting off or having sex with a partner.

4 Write your own erotic story and put you and your partner into the action. For even more fun, read it onto a tape and slip it into your lover's briefcase with a note to listen to it.

5 Go with your partner to a strip club and see if the atmosphere gets you in the mood for some one-on-one action. Go home and put on your own show for one another.

6 Take some erotic shots of yourself and send or give them to a partner with a note instructing him to meet you somewhere at a certain time to continue the adventure.

7 If you're an artist, have your partner pose naked for a drawing or painting.

Different forms of porn

Whatever form it takes, the purpose of porn is always the same: to stimulate us sexually. Whether that stimulation is an end in itself or leads to actual sexual activity, either alone or with someone else, is not really important. The point is that our senses have been stimulated, our minds and bodies have been engaged, and we've begun to explore what arouses us. When we understand what it is that gets us excited sexually, this naturally helps us to experience our erotic selves more fully and openly, even if this exploration never advances beyond the realm of fantasy.

One of the primary benefits of porn is that it allows us to explore our fantasies safely. Say, for example, you read an erotic story about a man engaged in a sexual experience that you've never encountered before, and perhaps you become unexpectedly aroused by it. Maybe you will actually explore the activity that's gotten you excited. Maybe you won't. The important thing is that you've allowed yourself to go there in your head, to experience something you might not have experienced otherwise.

Similarly, watching porn movies appeals to many men because it provides several forms of sexual stimulation. Watching men we find

PORNOGRAPHIC LITERATURE is something you can enjoy alone or with a partner. Reading pornographic magazines together can also be a form of foreplay.

Too much of a good thing

At what point does enjoying porn become enjoying it too much? When your sexual life revolves primarily around watching porn, reading porn, or searching for porn on the internet, it's time to look at what you're doing and why. It's possible that you're using pornography as a substitute for, rather than an enhancement of, sexual relationships with other people. So if you find yourself constantly using porn for sexual gratification, or unable to become sexually stimulated without it, it's time to throw out the magazines, turn off the TV, and get yourself out into the real world. If you find you need help doing this, consider contacting a support group for people dealing with sexual addiction.

attractive having sex can be enjoyable all on its own, whether we just watch or whether we stimulate ourselves physically as well. Some guys enjoy masturbating while watching porn, or perhaps using sex toys to simulate the action on the screen. Again, this can be a great way to explore your fantasies, or to play sexually during those times when you're either not involved with anyone else or when you're separated from a partner for some reason.

Coming together through porn

Even when you're partnered, you can use porn to enhance your sex life. Watching erotic videos with your lover provides an excellent opportunity for discussing what turns you on. Sometimes it can even create an opening for bringing up something you want to experience sexually but haven't known how to approach

your partner about trying. Some couples also enjoy recreating what the actors in porn films are doing, using porn as a sort of script to follow in their own lovemaking.

With all the different kinds of erotic materials available, it's important not to think of porn just as "dirty magazines" or as something you resort to when you can't get "the real thing." The expression of erotic desire is just as important as the expression of any other emotion, and allowing yourself to recognize and enjoy the many different expressions of sexuality can really enhance your sexual and emotional relationships. The important thing is to get away from notions of good and bad, to stop thinking of certain activities as being "dirty" or "wrong." When we can do that, we can really begin to explore who we are as sexual people.

Is it exploitation?

Not everyone finds pornography appealing or useful. While some of us may enjoy watching guys having sex on film or get off on seeing naked men in magazines, for others this is a turn-off. Many men who are in relationships feel that using porn for sexual gratification is degrading or disrespectful to their partner. It just depends on who you are and what you're comfortable with.

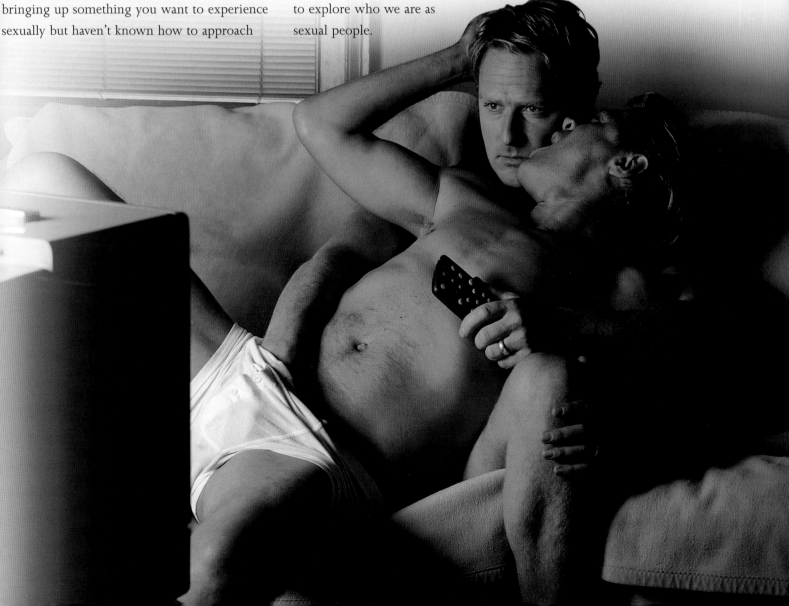

WATCHING PORNOGRAPHY TOGETHER can help to create a fun, sexy atmosphere and provide ideas to enhance your sexual repertoire.

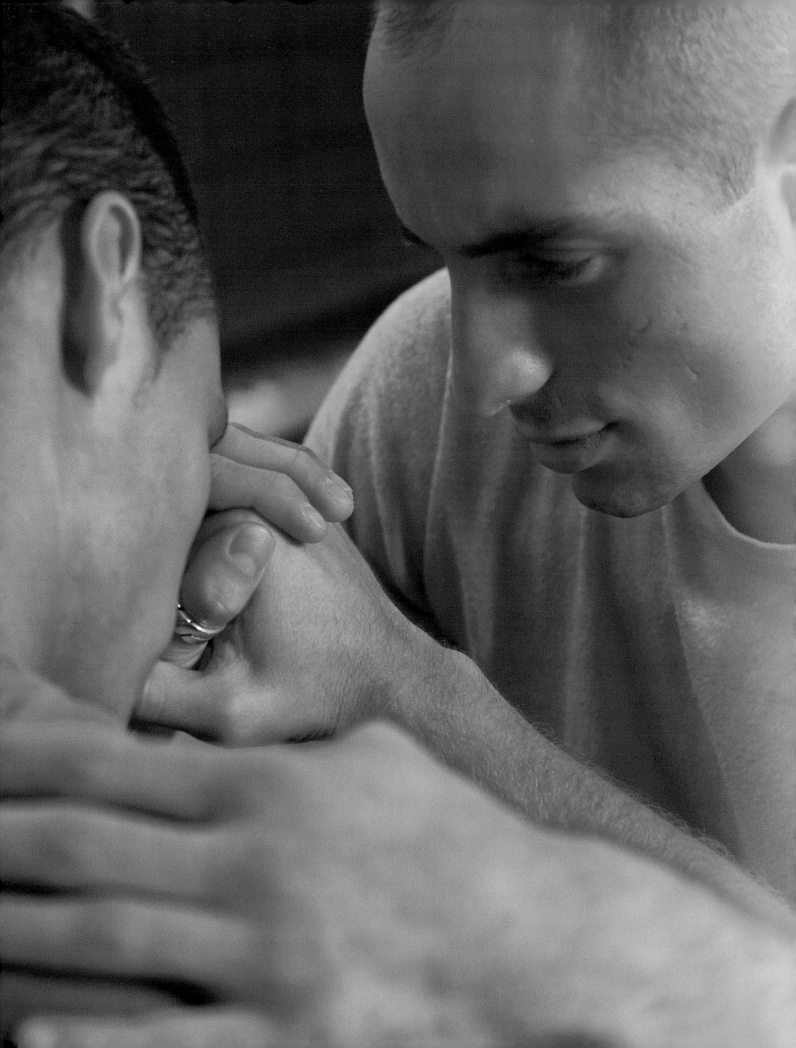

5 Problem solving

Exploring your sexuality is an exciting undertaking, and if you go about it with care, things should go smoothly. But from time to time you might encounter an obstacle or two, and when you do it's important to know how to deal with the situation. With a little planning, even the most troublesome problem can be handled thoughtfully and effectively.

When things go wrong

Dealing with issues

It would be great if sex were always perfect, always hot, always satisfying. But it isn't. From time to time we run into obstacles to sexual enjoyment. Some of these obstacles are physical or health-related, others are emotional or psychological. Sometimes we know what the problem is, but often we don't understand where the trouble is coming from. Whatever the cause or nature of issues in our sex lives, however, there are many ways to address and overcome them. By reading the next few pages you'll find out how to tackle some of these setbacks.

It's good to talk

It cannot be stressed too much or too often that the key to having good relationships and good sex is communication. When you are comfortable discussing issues with your partners, you're opening the door to being successful in establishing and maintaining satisfying and exciting relationships of all kinds. This is particularly true when you're dealing with potential obstacles to your sexual fulfilment. The same is true for problems that don't involve a partner, although in these cases the people you need to communicate with are yourself and any physicians, therapists, or counselors who might be involved. Again, listening to your own body,

It's like this, doc

It's seldom easy to talk to your doctor about sex-related issues. While it's unlikely that the doctor will be embarrassed, you may well be. You may even be fearful of disclosing information about your private life to someone you may barely know.

If you think that you won't feel comfortable talking to your general physician, make an appointment at a gay men's health center or a clinic that serves the gay community. Most large cities have them, and the doctors who work there are very familiar with the issues faced by gay men when it comes to sex. If you can't locate a doctor or clinic, ask the closest gay community center for a referral.

For general advice on problems encountered by gay men, see the list of resources and websites on pages 182–185.

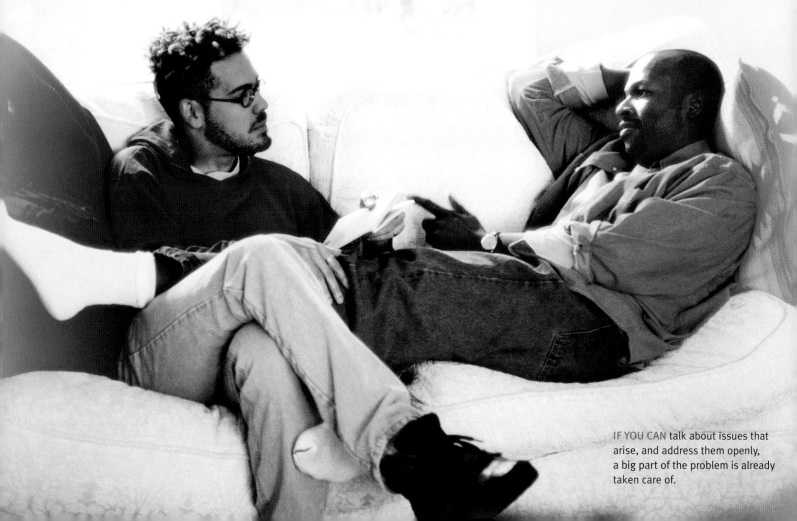

IF YOU CAN talk about issues that arise, and address them openly, a big part of the problem is already taken care of.

paying attention to your own needs, and creating an open dialogue with healthcare professionals will go a long way toward making treatment of sex-related issues a success.

Men's problems

Some common sex-related difficulties, challenges, and concerns encountered by men will be addressed in the next few pages, but it's important to remember that this is not a substitute for medical treatment or counseling: It is simply a discussion of problems that are commonly experienced, along with some general guidelines for handling them. If you are dealing with any sex-related issues, you will need more complete information and guidance from professional sources.

Before you can begin to address a problem you need to know that it exists. This seems obvious, but often it isn't. Not being able to attain erections is something you can identify easily, but how about a gradual loss of sex drive, or finding it more and more difficult to achieve orgasm? Often we ignore these situations, attributing them to other problems in our lives. Maybe they *are* related to other problems, but brushing them aside isn't going to make them go away.

It's important to note any changes in your sexual behavior or sexual performance—the first step in addressing issues. The second step is figuring out what to do about the problem. If the problem involves a partner, include him in discussions about it. Hoping he doesn't notice or that the problem will magically go away will only cause more problems. Your partner probably does notice and if nothing is said then you both might develop fears that could be eased if the concern were addressed directly.

If discussions with your partner aren't enough, then you will need to talk to professionals who have the knowledge and experience to help you. In this day and age, most doctors are well-trained in dealing with sex-related issues and, although talking about

personal issues with your physician might not be the most fun thing to do, it may be a necessary step. In some cases it may also be beneficial to speak with a counselor or therapist with experience in sex-related issues.

Working it out

Finally, having identified the problem, you need to treat it. If the trouble has something to do with your relationship with your partner, the two of you may have to work it out together, possibly with the aid of a counselor. If the problem is physical, you may need to address some health issues. Again, the important thing is that you listen, share, and remain aware of and open to the options available to you.

Good sex should be for life, and it can be. Maintaining an active, healthy sex life may mean making adjustments in other areas, but there's no reason why you can't remain actively and happily sexual for your whole life. Treat sex-related problems as you would any other health issues and you'll be well on your way to achieving that goal.

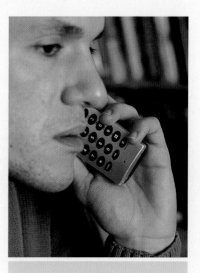

Time to talk

If your partner is the one who is experiencing sexual difficulties you may find yourself in a very uncomfortable position, particularly if he is reluctant to talk openly about what's happening. Most likely you'll want to help him, but at the same time you may be dealing with your own feelings of frustration, anxiety, or possibly even anger about the situation.

If your partner won't discuss the issue with you and is unwilling to seek help for the problem, you need to look for help for yourself. Don't simply confide in a friend. As much as this may relieve some of the stress, it may cause more problems if, for some reason, your partner finds out and thinks you've been sharing private information behind his back.

A better solution is to speak to a helpline, support group, or therapist on your own. Talking to someone who is not involved in your personal life will help you identify the various aspects of the problem, and then develop a plan for dealing with them.

It's important in situations such as these to remember that even though your partner is the one experiencing the problem, you are also greatly affected by it. Ignoring your own emotions and needs in an attempt to make him feel better will ultimately only make things worse for both of you.

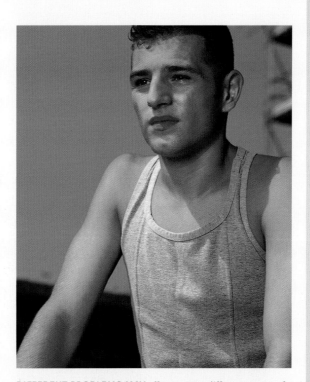

DIFFERENT PROBLEMS MAY affect men at different stages of their sexual lives. Most can be treated as long as you talk them through with your partner, friends, or a professional.

Erection problems

Stand up for yourself

One of the most common—and frustrating—problems related to sex is the evilly named "erectile dysfunction." Basically this means you have problems getting or maintaining erections. And although it's true that almost all of us experience this at some time, knowing that it happens to lots of other guys may not make it any less irritating. The good news is that most erection difficulties are relatively easy to deal with.

You're not alone

Just like the rest of your body, your penis is affected by your overall health, and erection difficulties are often a result of changes in your physical well-being. Long-term smokers and drinkers, for example, often experience decreased erections due to damage to the cardiovascular system. Aging also takes a toll

Keeping note

If you find yourself experiencing erection difficulties, it may help to keep a log of when (and with whom) they occur. If they continue over a period of time, you may be able to detect a pattern, such as an increase in occurrences during stressful times at work, or perhaps only with certain partners, or during specific types of sex.

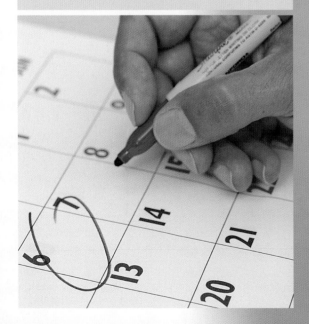

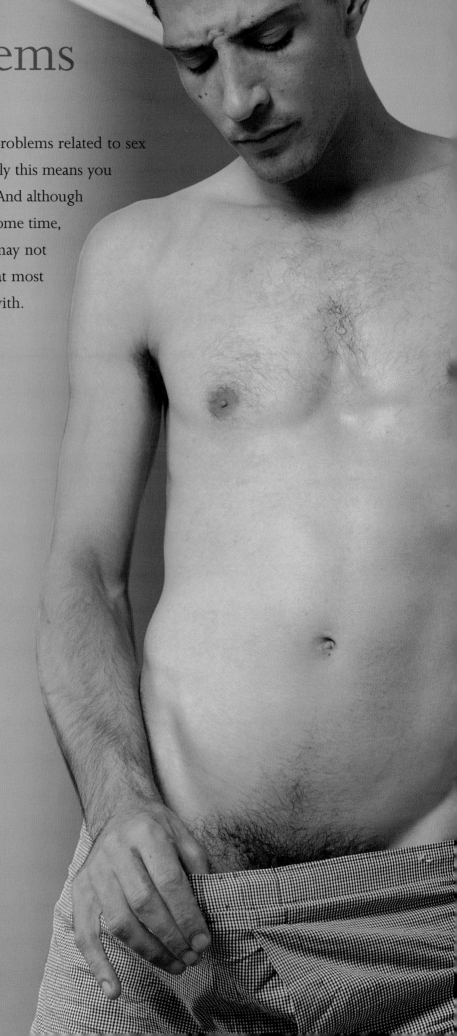

on the penis, and age-related conditions such as reduced testosterone levels and an enlarged prostate may affect erections. Many prescription medications and recreational drugs make it more difficult to get hard, stay hard, or reach orgasm.

Not surprisingly, erections can be influenced by psychological issues, notably depression and negative feelings about your body, your partner, your relationships, and sex in general. Even concerns at work can make arousal difficult.

So how do you know what the cause is? If your erection problems seem to come on suddenly and without discernible cause, it is likely to be physical. If they develop more gradually, it might be emotional. Your doctor will confirm or rule out most physical possibilities, and a therapist who specializes in sex-related issues can help pinpoint psychological barriers.

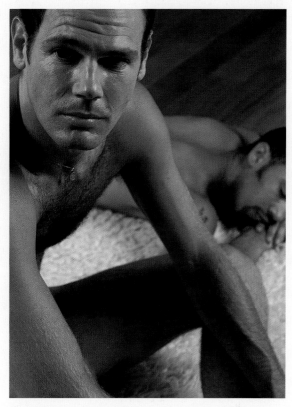

ADDRESSING THE PROBLEM of erectile dysfunction will ultimately be easier, more productive, and less stressful than just hoping it will go away on its own.

DISCUSSING ERECTION DIFFICULTIES with a partner may seem frightening or difficult, but not talking about it will only lead to more serious relationship problems.

Understanding the causes

It used to be thought that erectile dysfunction was primarily the result of psychological factors. We now know, however, that in many cases there is a physical cause to problems with achieving or maintaining erections, and often there is a combination of factors at work (see below). Major progress has been made in understanding and treating sexual dysfunction, and the majority of men who experience erectile difficulties can be successfully treated. If you experience these issues, begin by identifying and eliminating potential problems. Quit smoking, limit alcohol intake, and reduce stress and anxiety as much as possible. If this does not help, seek medical advice to determine if the cause is physical and consider consulting a counselor who specializes in sexual issues.

PHYSICAL CAUSES
Erectile dysfunction caused by physical factors often develops gradually and generally occurs during all sexual activities. Some of the most common physical causes include:

• Insufficient blood flow to the penis
• Excessive drainage of blood from he penis
• Damage or diseases affecting nerves in the penis
• Hormone imbalance
• Side effects of prescription drugs
• Alcohol and/or drug abuse
• Diabetes
• Heavy smoking
• High cholesterol
• Diseases affecting the erectile tissue of the penis
• Neurological diseases, stroke
• Severe chronic diseases such as kidney and liver failure

PSYCHOLOGICAL CAUSES
Erectile dysfunction caused by psychological factors often occurs suddenly, and frequently only during certain sexual activities or with particular partners. Although major psychological causes are usually easy to identify, often emotional causes for sexual issues are harder to pinpoint because they may not seem related to sexual problems. Common psychological causes of sexual dysfunction include:

• Stress and anxiety from work or home issues
• Partnership conflicts and dissatisfaction
• Depression
• Sexual boredom
• Unresolved sexual orientation

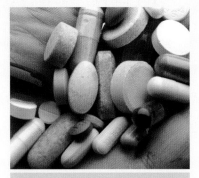

Too good to be true?

Beware of vitamins and supplements that claim to make your penis bigger or give you more sexual stamina. Most of them are simply loaded with stimulants such as caffeine, herbs, and other chemicals that increase blood flow. Although they may make you more energetic, some of them have been known to cause heart problems and even death. When it comes to your sexual health there are no magic formulas. Proper diet and exercise are your best bets. If you want to take supplements, do your research before trying anything.

The check-up

Looking after number one

Men, as a rule, don't go to the doctor very often. It probably has something to do with hating to ask for help and not looking forward to sitting on a cold exam table while people wearing latex gloves stick their hands in your crotch and order you to cough. Missing routine check-ups is one thing, but for gay men, not attending regular sexual check-ups is much more serious. Your doctor can detect little problems before they become really big problems, and knowing what's going on inside our bodies is part of maintaining healthy sex lives.

You're worth it

My father is one of those people who believes that if there's no visible blood and you can still walk upright then everything is fine, no matter how much it may hurt inside. This approach worked pretty well for him for 65 years, until all his brothers began dying of cancer and it was discovered that he himself had prostate cancer. Thankfully, they were able to treat him and he's fine, but he might have avoided a lot of the pain he ultimately went through had he gone to the doctor earlier.

I inherited his approach to health care, and after his diagnosis I went though a similar scare, when it was thought that a lump I discovered on one of my testicles (but had ignored for a year or two until my father's experience sent me

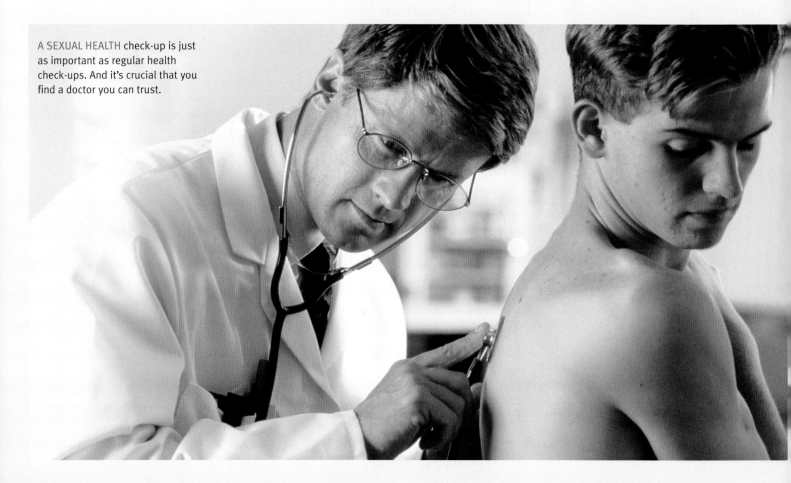

A SEXUAL HEALTH check-up is just as important as regular health check-ups. And it's crucial that you find a doctor you can trust.

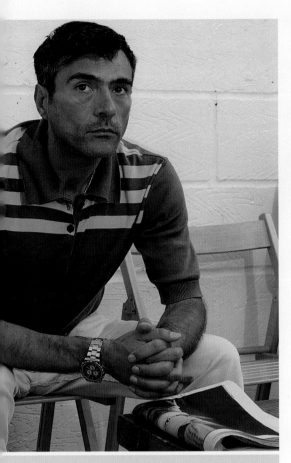

How often?

How often you need to have check-ups depends on your state of health. Most of us can get away with an annual check-up. But men with lots of sexual partners need more frequent visits. This is something you should definitely discuss with your doctor. The important thing is to get yourself there in the first place. If you've noticed changes in your health or in your body, you obviously want to get a check-up sooner rather than later. But even if you feel fine, set aside a day to have it done. It's one day, guys, and isn't it worth one day of boredom and unflattering paper-gown fashion to find out that everything's fine, instead of just hoping it is?

to the doctor), might actually be cancer. After numerous unpleasant tests, it was determined that it wasn't cancer after all, which was a relief, but I was annoyed at myself for waiting so long.

Very few of us like to take half the day to go pee in a cup, have our blood pressure taken, give blood, and be poked and prodded while a doctor busily takes notes. But here's the thing: Health stuff can just pop up out of the blue. Sometimes we don't have even the slightest clue

that something is going on inside. And the only way we're going to know is if we have someone poke around a little bit.

The essentials

As sexually active gay men there are some things we need to pay particular attention to. If you have multiple sexual partners, being tested for STDs (including HIV) is very important, particularly because many of them don't have obvious symptoms and you could be doing yourself and your partners a lot of damage by leaving them untreated. Testing for diseases such as hepatitis is also recommended. Men who engage in anal sex want to be sure that they're checked for any possible rectal problems (particularly hemorrhoids and tears). And of course all men need to be aware of the potential problems associated with the prostate.

Finding the right doctor

Along with a general dislike of going to the doctor, gay men have another potential obstacle to face when it comes to health. Many of us don't feel comfortable talking with our doctors about sexual matters. A lot of us don't have regular doctors and without an ongoing relationship it's not always easy to determine whether or not we can talk openly about our sex lives and our health. Yes, we *should* be able to. But sometimes we can't, or think that we can't.

One way around this, of course, is to find a gay doctor or a doctor who works extensively with gay patients. Then you know that you can talk about anything, and the doctor will be both knowledgeable and nonjudgmental. But this isn't always an option. In that case, you need to find a doctor you feel comfortable with. You can do this by asking friends who they go to, but again, you might be limited in your choices by your health insurance or other factors. If the doctor you're seeing responds negatively to your questions or makes you feel uncomfortable discussing your sexuality, find another one.

Do it yourself

There's one important health-related thing that you can and should do for yourself, and that's a testicular self-exam. It's easy to do, and it may help you detect potential problems early on.

You should do your self-exam regularly—maybe on the first day of every month.

To examine your testicles, simply hold them in your hands and, one at a time, gently feel them all over with your thumb and fingers. It's particularly easy to do this in the shower or after bathing, when the skin is warm and the scrotum is relaxed so you can feel its contents easily. Soaping the scrotum can also make self-examinations easier.

What you're looking for are any changes in size or texture, in particular small lumps and swellings. All men have some bumpiness on the testicles where the epididymis (structures for holding sperm) attach to them. What you want to be aware of are any unusual bumps, particularly if they're painful or seem to be getting larger.

This self-exam is a very easy thing to do, and can help detect any signs of testicular cancer, which, fortunately, is one of the most easily and effectively treated forms of cancer when detected early on. By routinely performing a check on yourself, you'll come to know what your testicles normally look and feel like, and will be able to detect any changes should they occur. If you do notice any changes, consult your doctor straightaway—if you don't, you may worry needlessly.

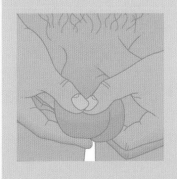

Types of STDs

Recognizing and treating sex-related diseases

Sexually transmitted diseases (STDs) are a very real concern for men who have sex with men. Unfortunately, apart from AIDS, we often don't think or talk about STDs. They're not exactly sexy (even the names are ugly), and we don't like to dwell on the idea that the hot body we're enjoying so intimately might be concealing something potentially unpleasant. But the fact is that a large percentage of us *do* harbor various bacteria and viruses, and we can pass these things to one another during sexual activity. So let's address STDs and find out a little more about them.

Knowledge is power

Knowing what the different STDs are, what their symptoms are, and how they can be passed on from person to person is important. Fortunately, most (but not all) STDs can be treated fairly easily, as long as they're caught early on. This doesn't mean we can afford to have a casual attitude about them, however. Some STDs (such as AIDS and hepatitis) are extremely damaging to the body. Even more common STDs (such as herpes) can affect our sexual behavior for the rest of our lives. And contracting any STD at all is, at best, irritating and disruptive to our sex lives. So take them seriously.

The chart shown on page 168–169 details the most common STDs encountered by gay men. As you'll see, many STDs have similar symptoms, so don't assume you can correctly identify a possible STD just by this information. If you think you might have contracted something, you need to have yourself examined by a doctor. If you don't feel comfortable visiting your regular doctor, cities with sizable gay populations usually have health clinics familiar with STDs common to gay men.

When we think about STDs, we sometimes associate them with dirty people or sexual acts that are somehow out of the ordinary. In short, we think of people who aren't us, and this is wrong. The reality is that STDs have little to do with how clean you are, what kind of sex you

have, or what kind of person you are. They are simply diseases, infections, and parasites. They can be transmitted to anyone, by anyone, in many different kinds of situations.

We're all targets

It's important that we don't think of STDs as something to be ashamed of or as things that only happen to certain sections of society. All of us who engage in sex with other people can potentially be affected by an STD. You should remember that they are a health issue, not a reflection of someone's character or a gauge of a person's trustworthiness.

And what exactly is an STD? We call them sexually transmitted diseases because they can be passed from one person to another during sexual behavior. That behavior is not limited to intercourse. It can include *any* behavior involved with sex, from kissing and fondling to oral sex, and in some cases even simply rubbing against someone. So when you think about STDs, don't just think about the genitals. Consider the full range of sexual expression.

The majority of STDs are, in fact, spread through contact with the genitals or the rectum. This contact can involve the penis, mouth, or fingers. Transmission occurs when these body parts come into contact with a partner's infected areas (or also via sex toys that have been used on infected areas), or when a bacteria or virus contained in semen, blood, or feces comes into contact with a partner. Certain external parasites, such as crab lice and scabies, can be spread simply by rubbing against a partner who is infested with them.

Weighing the risks

Because of these various means of transmission, it is very important to understand the risks of your sexual behaviors. For example, the STD gonorrhea can be present in the penis, the rectum, and the throat. Unprotected sex can not only spread the infection from one partner to another, but also from one part of the body to another. Similarly, inserting the fingers into the rectum and then using them elsewhere without washing first can easily spread parasites such as giardia and shigella bacteria.

I'm not trying to create a portrait of the body as a minefield; I simply want you to be aware of how easy it is to pass STDs back and forth. Knowing what *can* happen doesn't mean it will happen; it just means that you will be better educated and better equipped to make decisions about your sexual health.

Knowing when you might have been infected with an STD is crucial. Some things, such as crabs, are pretty obvious because you see and feel them. But other STDs can be much more difficult to recognize, primarily because a lot of their symptoms are similar. In general, you should be on the lookout for anything that looks or feels unusual.

The telltale signs

Knowing what to look out for means being prepared. Start with your penis. If you feel burning or stinging when you urinate, or if you suddenly notice any kind of discharge from your penis or stains appearing on your underwear for no apparent reason, you should be concerned. Many STDs result in a whitish discharge. This may or may not be accompanied

by redness, soreness, scabs, or bumps on the penis. Some STDs affecting the rectum also result in bumps, discharge, and soreness in that area.

By remaining aware of what your body normally looks and feels like, you'll be more likely to notice when something has changed. Conduct regular examinations of your penis and your rectum. If you notice anything unusual, check it out. It may turn out to be nothing, but you want to be sure. If left unchecked, many STDs can cause extensive damage to the body, and because some STDs seem to go away on their own but are really still operating inside your body, it's important to have yourself tested even if the symptoms lessen or go away.

A sense of perspective

If it turns out that you do have an STD, it's not the end of the world. It may mean making some lifestyle changes, but in most cases STDs are only temporary inconveniences. In the meantime, avoid all sexual contact with other people until you are either free of the STD or until it is not possible to spread it to anyone else. Even STDs that have a long-range effect on your health (hepatitis, herpes, and HIV, for example) don't mean the end of your sex life. Again, the key is early detection and treatment, which is why knowing everything you can about STDs is so important.

Equally important is knowing how to prevent STDs in the first place. You can't completely eliminate the possibility of being affected by an STD unless you never have sex. Even asking a partner if he has an STD isn't foolproof because many people have them and don't even know it. But by following safer sex practices, you will eliminate many of the opportunities for infection with an STD, and by keeping a close eye on your own sexual health you will be able to take the necessary steps, should you ever be exposed to one.

Protect yourself against contracting STDs by educating yourself about them and by always practicing safer sex with your partners.

What to do if you have an STD

If you suspect that you have contracted an STD, the most important thing to do is not panic. Many STDs are easily treatable, particularly when caught early on, and even the most serious STDs do not have to be life-threatening.

• Get tested. The longer you wait, the more damage the STD may do. If you even suspect that you have been exposed to an STD, it's important to be tested.

• Tell your partners. If you know the person from whom you contracted the STD, make sure you tell him (he might not even be aware that he has it.) Let any other recent sexual partners know so that they can have themselves tested as well. What's important is making sure it doesn't spread to anyone else.

• If you have an STD that cannot be eradicated completely (such as genital herpes), learn how to discuss the situation with any future partners.

• Practice good personal hygiene to avoid transferring infections to other parts of your body or to others through casual contact.

A—Z OF CONDITIONS

What follows is a listing of the STDs that most commonly affect gay men. If you think you may have been exposed to an STD, you need to have yourself tested to determine the exact cause, because many STDs have similar symptoms.

AIDS

AIDS is caused by HIV, a virus passed from partner to partner sexually through infected blood and semen. See more information on pages 170–173.

SYMPTOMS: Symptoms of HIV infection vary and can be very similar to symptoms of the flu. Often more severe symptoms don't appear until later stages of infection. For this reason, regular testing for HIV is recommended.

TESTING: Blood test.

TREATMENT: There is currently no cure for HIV infection. Improved treatments are ensuring longer, healthier lives for HIV-positive people, but the virus still takes a terrible toll on the body.

Chlamydia

Chlamydia is caused by bacteria that spread from partner to partner when mucous membranes (particularly in the rectum) come into contact with infected semen. Untreated, it can lead to inflammation of the prostate and/or epididymis, scarring of the urethra, and infertility.

SYMPTOMS: Discharge from penis or anus. Possible pain during urination. Symptoms appear 1–3 weeks after infection and then disappear. Fifty percent of men have no symptoms.

TESTING: Tests on urine or genital discharge.

TREATMENT: Antibiotics.

Crabs and Scabies

Crabs are very small bugs that attach themselves to pubic hair (where they lay their eggs) and bite the surrounding skin. Scabies are mites that dig under the skin around the genital area, where they lay their eggs. Crabs and mites are transmitted from body-to-body contact and also through infested clothing, sheets, and bedding.

SYMPTOMS: Itching, bumps, and visible bugs.

TESTING: Sight.

TREATMENT: Over-the-counter and prescription solutions. Shaving the hair from affected areas may also help, because it eliminates holdfasts and removes any eggs attached to the hair. All bedding, towels, and clothing must be washed in hot water and dried on a high setting to kill remaining bugs and eggs.

Giardia, Amebiasis, Cryptosporidium

Similar to shigella, these three parasites are spread through oral-anal contact (rimming), through oral contact with contaminated fingers or toys, and through oral contact with contaminated skin. They can also be passed on in water infected with fecal material. The parasites reside in the intestines (occasionally migrating to the liver), where they result in diarrhea, cramping, and general discomfort.

SYMPTOMS: Stomach cramps and diarrhea.

TESTING: Examination of stool.

TREATMENT: Antibiotics.

Gonorrhea

A bacterial infection spread through anal and/or oral sex with a partner infected in his throat or anus. It can be spread from the anus to the throat and vice versa.

SYMPTOMS: Symptoms generally develop within 2–5 days of infection, but may take up to 30 days. They include white discharge from the penis or anus, pain or itching in the head of the penis, swelling of the penis or testicles, pain or burning during urination, frequent urination, anal or rectal itching, and pain during bowel movements. Gonorrhea of the throat often has no symptoms, except possibly a sore throat.

TESTING: Tests on urine or genital discharge.

TREATMENT: Antibiotics.

Hepatitis A, B, and C

A virus that causes inflammation of the liver, liver failure, liver cancer, and, in some cases, death. Hepatitis A is spread through contaminated water, food, and stool (making oral-anal contact a mode of transmission). Hepatitis B is spread through contact with infected semen or blood. Hepatitis C is usually transmitted through shared needles or from blood transfusions, but infection through sex (where blood is present) is also possible.

SYMPTOMS: Symptoms vary greatly, and might not appear at all. They can include fatigue, stomach pain, yellowing of the skin or eyes, dark urine, light-colored stool, and fever.

TESTING: Blood test.

TREATMENT: Vaccinations are available for A and B. There is no vaccination for Hepatitis C. Treatment for all forms of hepatitis is bed rest and time. It can take months or even years to recover from it, so prevention is very important. Although hepatitis usually clears up by itself, it is possible to develop chronic hepatitis. This means that the virus will remain in the body for many

...ears. While people with chronic hepatitis do not generally suffer continually from it while infected, there is the possibility that they may be able to infect others with the virus, so safer sex precautions should be followed.

Herpes

A viral infection transmitted via skin-to-skin contact during sex. Herpes is unusual in that once it's in your system it remains there forever and can be passed on to your partners even if no symptoms are present. The presence of herpes sores makes it three to five times more likely that HIV will be contracted if it's present.

SYMPTOMS: Maybe none. When present, symptoms appear as blisters or sores which turn into scabs and fall off. Swollen glands, fever, and body aches may also be present.

TESTING: Generally diagnosed by sight. Blood tests and viral culture tests using fluid from a sore are also used.

TREATMENT: There is currently no cure for herpes, although there are several medications used to reduce the severity of outbreaks.

HPV

The human papillomavirus (HPV) is the virus that causes genital warts, sometimes called condyloma. It is passed via skin-to-skin contact during anal sex. HPV is thought to be the most common STD, with some studies estimating that 95% of HIV-positive men and 65% of HIV-negative men have it. There are many different types of HPV, most of them harmless, but some may cause changes in the cells of the anus, leading to cancer.

SYMPTOMS: HPV forms wart-like bumps on the penis and/or around the rectum, which are generally painless but sometimes itchy.

TESTING: Examination of genital warts. Anal pap smears. Biopsy.

TREATMENT: There is no treatment for HPV. The virus lives in your body forever. Warts may be removed by a physician using various means. Over-the-counter wart removers should never be used on genital warts.

Molluscum Contagiosum

It sounds like something out of *Harry Potter*, but actually this is a viral disease that causes small, harmless but ugly, tumors or lesions to appear on your skin. It can be passed via skin-to-skin contact, which is why it's considered an STD.

SYMPTOMS: Approximately 4-12 weeks after exposure to the virus, pin-sized growths resembling pimples appear, generally in the area of the genitals, buttocks, abdomen, and lower thighs. These pimples are usually firm, shiny, and pink, white, or flesh-colored, and may have a crater-like depression in the center. (Sometimes this indentation appears only after the lesions become more developed.) The growths slowly increase in size, eventually becoming the size of a pea. They may or may not appear in clusters, although there are usually multiple lesions.

TESTING: Sight.

TREATMENT: The molloscum contagiosum virus cannot be killed, but will usually disappear within a few months. The lesions themselves can be removed by a physician.

Shigella

A bacterial infection spread through oral-anal contact (rimming), through oral contact with contaminated fingers or toys, and through oral contact with contaminated skin.

SYMPTOMS: Stomach cramps and diarrhea.

TESTING: Examination of stool.

TREATMENT: Antibiotics.

Syphilis

Syphilis is a bacterial infection spread by physical contact during anal or oral sex. Untreated, it can cause organ and brain damage. It also makes HIV easier to catch or transmit.

SYMPTOMS: Symptoms occur in four stages. Stage one (Primary) occurs 2–12 weeks after exposure and appears as a skin sore that may be on the scrotum, penis, or anus, or inside the anus or mouth. Stage two (Secondary) develops 4–12 weeks after infection and appears as a skin rash on the palms and soles of the feet. Swollen glands, fever, fatigue, patchy hair loss, weight loss, and headache are also sometimes present. There also may be syphilis warts and white patches in the mouth or anus. Stage three (Latent) has no symptoms, and at this stage the infection can be detected only by a blood test. If untreated, the syphilis advances to Stage four (Tertiary) in which damage to internal organs (usually the brain, heart, liver, and bones) can occur, resulting in paralysis, mental problems, blindness, deafness, heart failure, and death.

TESTING: Blood test.

TREATMENT: Antibiotics.

HIV and AIDS

The story so far

In the early 1980s, the first cases of what was then called "gay cancer" were reported. As the number of people with the disease increased at a staggering rate, it went through several name changes until the medical community settled on AIDS—Acquired Immune Deficiency Syndrome. What was once believed to be an illness affecting only a handful of people became one of the largest epidemics the world has ever known. It also became a social and political issue that galvanized the gay community, increasing awareness of gay health issues, and changing forever the way gay men think about sex.

Back to the drawing board

Those of us who lived through the height of the AIDS epidemic will never forget the toll it took on our community. Unfortunately, in the wake of improved treatment for people with AIDS, some of us seem to be forgetting what we learned about how HIV, the virus that causes AIDS, is and is not transmitted. Owing to this form of sexual amnesia, in recent years new cases of HIV infection have been rising at an alarming rate, particularly among young men, suggesting that a new wave of the epidemic is coming. Once again, understanding what AIDS is, what it does, and how it can be prevented is of utmost importance to us as a community of sexually active men.

The basics are simple enough to understand. AIDS is caused by HIV, a virus similar to the viruses that cause other diseases such as colds and flus. Once HIV has infiltrated the body, it attacks the immune system, destroying it until the infected person is unable to fight off infections and dies as a result. Unlike cold and flu viruses, however, HIV cannot be transmitted through casual contact (such as by sneezing or sharing cups). It must come into direct contact with the blood in order to infect. How does it do this? In three main ways: through sexual contact, through the use of shared needles to inject drugs or steroids, and through blood transfusions with infected blood (a very rare occurrence today). That's it. Three ways.

Because contracting HIV through sexual contact is the form of transmission most gay men are concerned about, let's look at various sexual activities and see how they relate to HIV infection.

Anal and oral sex—the risks

Engaging in anal sex is the primary means of HIV transmission in gay men. The rectum is composed of a delicate membrane. This membrane can be scraped or torn for many reasons, including penetration with a finger or dildo, or from excessive douching (which dries out the membrane). It's also possible for the membrane to be scraped or torn by the friction of the penis rubbing against it during anal sex. When semen from an infected partner is ejaculated into the rectum, the AIDS virus (which is found in semen as well as blood) can enter the recipient's bloodstream through the compromised membrane.

Oral sex provides a similar route of transmission. Cuts on the gums, tongue, or any part of the mouth, may provide direct entry into the bloodstream for a virus contained in semen, and which is ejaculated into the mouth. The transmission of HIV through oral sex is one of the most debated issues in regard to AIDS. We know that transmision *can* occur during oral sex, but we don't know how often this has actually been the case. Many researchers

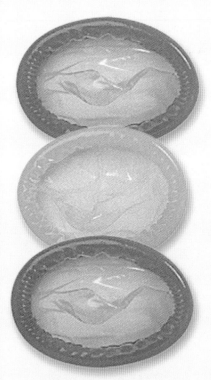

WHEN USED PROPERLY, latex condoms provide the most effective protection against the spread of HIV.

consider it a relatively low-risk activity, but low-risk does not mean no risk, so understand that this is a potential means of transmission.

In discussing both the anal and oral transmission of HIV, we've focused on the passive partner, meaning the partner who is receiving the active partner's penis (and therefore the semen) into his rectum or mouth. It's true that the receptive partner is at greater risk for contracting HIV than the active partner is. But there is also associated risk with putting your penis into someone else's rectum or mouth. This is because infected blood in your partner's rectum or mouth could come into contact with any scrapes, cuts, or sores on your penis. Again, the likelihood of transmission through these routes is low, but it is still a possibility.

Preventing infection

Many myths surround the subject of HIV and how it can and cannot be killed. Although it's true that the virus lives for only a short time outside the body, it's not true that it is killed by nonoxynol-9, the spermicide commonly applied to condoms as a pregnancy preventative. Nor is infection prevented by rinsing your mouth with alcohol or mouthwash before or after oral sex, or by douching after anal sex. In short, killing HIV is not a form of protection: only using barriers during sex is. This message is simple enough to understand—putting it into practice is the hard part.

Okay, so you understand what HIV and AIDS are and are not, but what does it all mean? Put simply, it means you need to know how to prevent transmission of HIV during sex, and that means using barriers between yourself and your partner's semen or between yourself and your partner's blood. The most effective barrier is a latex condom (not lambskin, which can allow HIV to pass through). When used properly this provides the greatest measure of protection. It's an easy equation to get your head around: If infected semen or blood can't reach your bloodstream, you can't become infected.

Knowing the risks of various sexual activities, it's up to you to decide what you are and are not comfortable doing. To learn more, take a look at some of the books and websites listed on pages 182–185. What you decide to do with this information is up to you. No one can, or should, make decisions about your health except you.

take a look at some of the books and websites listed on pages 182–185.

Prevention tips

Follow these guidelines to practicing safe sex and you'll keep the risk of contracting HIV to a minimum.

• Don't floss or brush your teeth right before oral sex: It can cause bleeding of the gums and mouth.

• Keep your fingernails trimmed to prevent cutting your partner during anal penetration with your fingers.

• Don't assume that pulling out before ejaculation will prevent transmission. HIV is found in precum as well as semen.

• Don't simply trust your partner to pull out. We all get carried away sometimes.

• Don't wear two condoms at once. This can actually cause tears because of the extra friction.

• A condom cut down the middle and spread over the anus can act as a barrier during oral-anal sex.

• Remove penis piercings before putting on a condom because they can cause tears.

• Don't assume you can tell if a guy has HIV by how he looks. You can't.

Why isn't there a cure for AIDS?

Although the scientific community is making great gains in AIDS treatment and prevention, a proven vaccine has been elusive. This is due primarily to the nature of HIV, the virus that causes AIDS. Both remarkable and frightening for its ability to change and survive in the face of new treatments, the virus is able to mutate, creating new strains that are resistant to formerly effective treatments. This makes finding a universally viable vaccination almost impossible—for the time being, at least.

Essentially, HIV works by invading the white blood cells of an infected person and tricking those cells into producing copies of the AIDS virus rather than copies of themselves, as they normally would do. In this way, HIV multiplies quickly while simultaneously destroying the cells it occupies and crippling the immune system. This in turn leaves the infected person susceptible to the opportunistic infections that are most often the cause of death in persons with AIDS.

Does this mean that the HIV virus is unstoppable? No. Someday there will be both a cure and a preventative. But until then it means that educating ourselves, practicing safer sex, and maintaining a high level of personal responsibility are the best defenses against the disease.

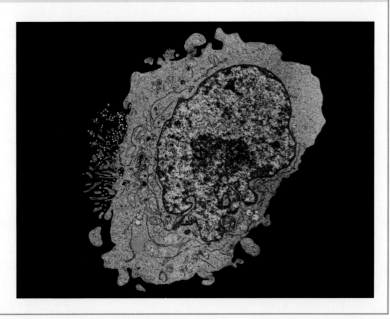

Living with HIV

Taking responsibility for yourself

In the early days of the AIDS crisis, testing positive for HIV was essentially a death sentence. Treatments were almost nonexistent and, because we didn't really know how to control the disease, it almost always meant that the infected person would die within a relatively short time. More than 20 years since HIV was first recognized, there remains no vaccine against HIV and no cure for AIDS, but thanks to years of research we've developed many different treatments for people with HIV infection. Today, people living with the virus are enjoying longer, healthier lives.

Making the adjustment

For a long time people living with HIV infection assumed that a positive diagnosis meant the end of their sex lives, or at least having their sex lives severely limited. Thanks to scientific research and subsequent education, we now know that doesn't have to be the case. HIV-positive men are simply people living with a virus. Being HIV-positive, or being with an HIV-positive partner, means having to adjust your thinking and your behavior in certain ways, but it doesn't have to limit your sexual expression or enjoyment.

There are two components to sexual relationships and the HIV status of the partners involved: a physical component and an emotional component. The health issues are simple to address, so we'll discuss these first.

If you are a man living with HIV, your immune system is compromised to some degree. As a result of this, you may be more susceptible to becoming infected with any viruses your partners may have. And this means infections that an uncompromised immune system might easily fight off may not be fought off by your body. So it's important for you to know the status of your own health, and to take whatever precautions are necessary to keep yourself as healthy as possible.

If you are HIV-negative, of course you have the issue of remaining uninfected. Being HIV-negative means understanding safer-sex techniques and making sure you practice them.

More tricky to handle are the emotional aspects of HIV infection and how it affects attitudes toward sex. Some men, fearing that they will become infected with HIV, stop having sex altogether. Others, feeling that becoming infected is inevitable, choose to ignore safer-sex guidelines and risk infection. Men who are HIV-positive may also choose to stop having sex or to go to the opposite extreme and have as much sex as possible because they feel they have nothing to lose by doing so.

None of these attitudes are healthy ones. What is healthy is accepting AIDS as a fact of life for us as gay men. And that doesn't mean we have to let it control our sex lives. It means that we have to be educated, responsible people, and that we may have to be willing to make some compromises when it comes to our sexual relationships.

Taking precautionary measures

As with many sex-related issues, one of the biggest concerns associated with HIV is how to talk about it. Men who are HIV-positive wonder how, when, and even if they should tell potential partners. Men who aren't positive wonder how and when they should ask partners about their status.

There are no easy answers to this. Sure, it would be great if we could always talk freely about all sex-related issues. It would be wonderful if we could always trust our partners to be honest about everything. It would be fantastic if we all cared about each other's health as much as we care about our own. But life isn't like that, especially when it comes to sex, and especially when it comes to sex that occurs in the heat of passion, when the last thing on your mind is asking your partner what his HIV status is.

The safest course of action is to assume that every partner you have could be HIV-positive and to act accordingly. Even if you ask a partner about his status, he could be positive and not know it, or for some reason he could be uncomfortable about telling you the truth. By assuming that all your partners are potentially HIV-positive and practicing safer sex with all of them, you create a situation where asking isn't important because the opportunity for infection isn't there.

For HIV-positive men there are additional issues. If you fear being rejected by a partner because of your HIV status, discussing the issue may be the last thing you want to do. Also, you may feel pressure to be the responsible one and bring up the issue of safer sex. Again, if you act as if all your partners could be positive and insist that they do the same, the issue of your own status doesn't need to be discussed directly unless you want to. Of course, if you plan on a more serious relationship with a partner then it is something you will want, and need, to discuss at some point. Instead of worrying about any of these issues, remember that the more you know about HIV the less you have to fear.

LIVING WITH HIV may bring some changes to your life, but it doesn't change who you are as a person, as a man, or as a partner.

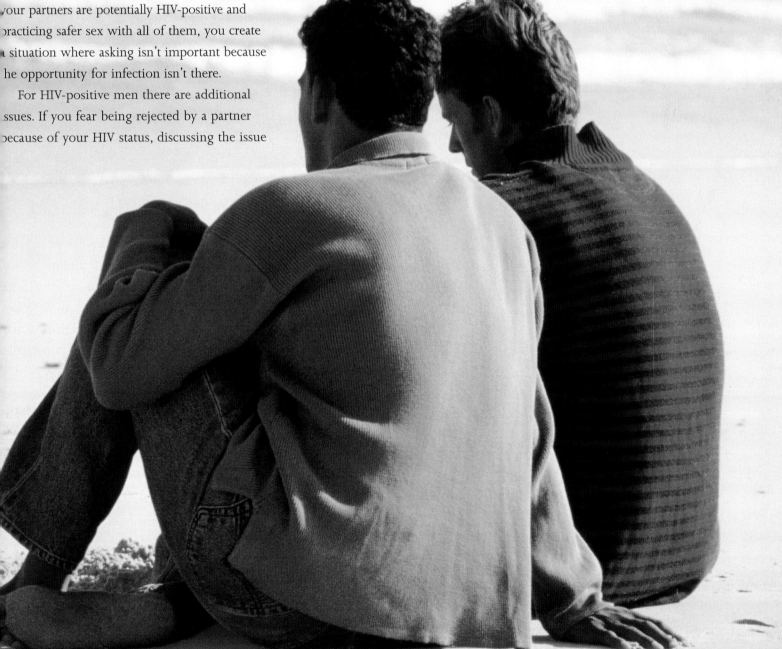

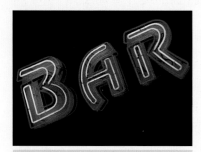

Alcohol and sex

A heady cocktail

For many people alcohol plays an integral role in social life. Bars, clubs, and parties all provide opportunities for spending time with friends and meeting potential partners, and alcohol is frequently used as a way to relax, to lessen our fears about talking to people, and to create feelings of well-being. This is all well and good, but when alcohol use is taken to the extreme it can create a number of problems. Knowing how alcohol affects the body is important to establishing your own rules for alcohol use and for understanding its potential for harm.

Drinking and dating

Most of us have had a beer or cocktail to unwind after work or to relax on a date or on a night out with the guys. Maybe a glass of wine or a vodka and tonic helps us to stop obsessing for a while about the stresses we're experiencing in other areas of our lives, or allows us to get into the mood of a party or bar crowd. Whatever the reason, it generally works, because alcohol acts as a depressant, interfering with the messages being sent back and forth in the

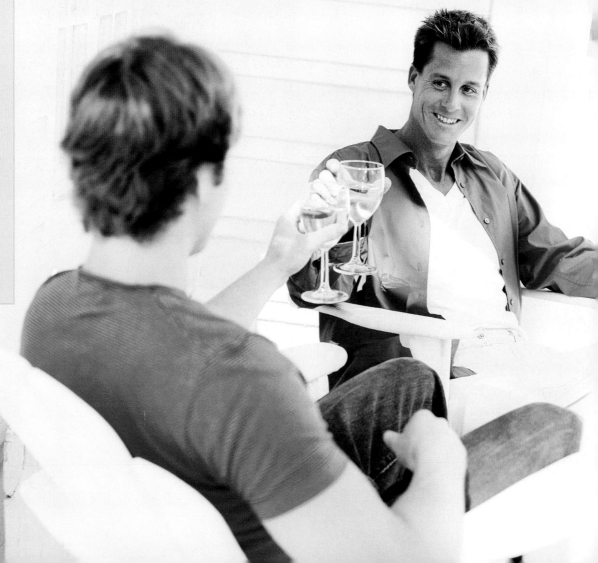

DRINKING SOCIALLY and in moderation can help you relax, feel more self-confident, and make the conversation flow.

brain—messages that can tell us to be anxious, angry, or tense. In effect, alcohol slows down the neural pathways and makes it more difficult for anxiety-producing communications to get through successfully.

This dulling of the senses isn't always a bad thing. Some men find that a drink or two helps them overcome feelings of anxiety associated with being in social settings. Downing a beer or having a shot of whiskey allows some of us to let down our guard a little and begin to enjoy being around other people or in settings—loud bars, for example, or crowded parties—where we might otherwise be irritable or tense and unable to have a good time. We may find that alcohol can allow us to explore desires and interests we might feel hesitant about when our anxieties get in the way.

More than just Dutch courage

But it's important to remember that even when alcohol is having a positive effect, it is in some measure an artificial effect. Even when drinking brings out something good in you or makes you feel more confident or relaxed, your reactions and responses are still altered. This means that you might behave in ways you wouldn't when you're not under the influence of alcohol.

Alcohol impairs judgment. Under its spell you may hook up with people you wouldn't consider otherwise, do things you wouldn't do when totally sober, or just behave in ways you might be embarrassed about later. Again, letting your defenses down a bit might not be a bad thing, but when you let them down so far that you engage in behavior you're not so happy about later on, it's a problem.

When it comes to sex, alcohol also has some physical effects. Too much alcohol in the system can make it difficult to have an erection or reach orgasm. More importantly, it can make you more likely to engage in sexual behavior that might not be the safest. And, in general, alcohol abuse contributes to all kinds of health issues,

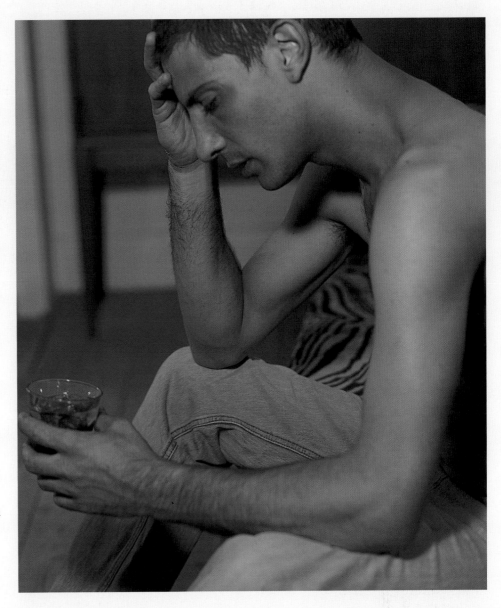

HUNG OVER Drinking too much alcohol can lead to unsafe sexual behavior that puts your health at risk and causes a wide range of emotional issues, including depression.

from liver and kidney damage to obesity and digestive problems. In addition, alcohol often interacts with medications and recreational drugs, magnifying or negating their effects, so it's imperative to know whether anything you're taking is affected by alcohol use.

So go ahead, let your hair down and have the occasional drink. But stay in control. Knowing what your own limits are will help you make decisions about when to drink, how much you should drink, and what to do when you've had too much.

Drunk and more drunk

The effects of alcohol can initially create a feeling of happiness, but when too much alcohol is consumed these feelings often reverse and turn into ones of depression, anger, or even fear. Drinking to forget, or to improve a negative mood, often results in the very things you're trying to avoid: obsessing over problems, becoming enraged, and lashing out at people. When these moods set in, it's often difficult to realize what's happening, and it's too late to stop them. So drink in moderation.

Domestic violence

Signs, symptoms, and solutions

We all get angry. We all fight with our partners from time to time. But sometimes things can go too far and someone can get hurt. Domestic violence—both physical and emotional—is as much a problem in the gay community as it is in the larger community. Unfortunately, it's not something we talk about very much. But we should, because the damage that can be done through emotional and physical abuse can be devastating, and it can take a long time to recover from it. So understanding what abuse is, and how to deal with it, is important for all of us.

Does no mean no?

Yep, no *does* mean no. Date rape doesn't just happen to young women. If you find yourself in a situation where someone has forced you to engage in sex you did not consent to, you don't have to keep quiet about it. Call your local gay community or health center first, discuss the situation, and if you want to take things further, contact the police.

Varieties of violence

When we think of domestic violence we usually imagine someone being hauled away by police after beating a partner. And in the most obvious examples of abuse this is true: Someone gets hit and winds up with bruises, broken bones, or worse. But violence isn't always that obvious, and abuse doesn't always leave bruises.

Unkind words, controlling behavior, and subjecting a partner to emotional "punishment" are also forms of abuse. If he says he can't live without you, or that if you leave he'll do something terrible to himself or to you, this is abuse. Constantly spying or accusing a partner of cheating when there's no basis for suspicion is abuse, as is using past infidelity or other behavior as a weapon in emotional battles. So is stealing from a partner or using joint finances to fund a drug addiction or gambling problem.

When push comes to shove

In short, abuse is any behavior that causes ongoing or severe emotional or physical pain for a partner. Getting into a fight and saying something we later regret is not necessarily abuse unless it's something done to control someone. Pushing a partner away when you're angry and don't want him to touch you is not

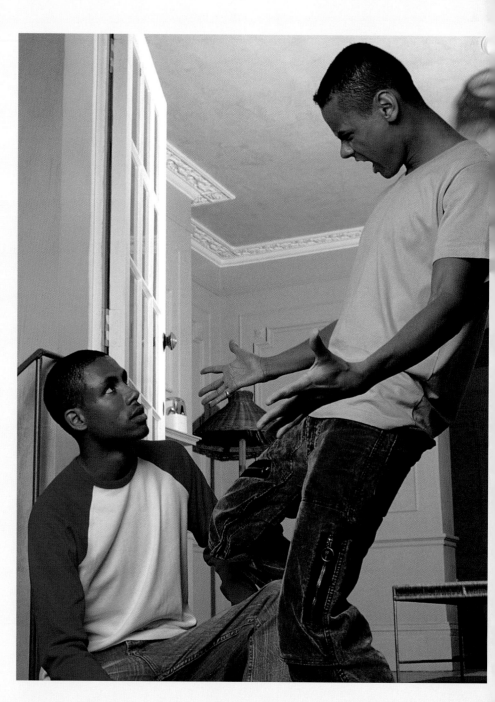

LEARNING TO CONTROL your anger is crucial to the prevention of domestic violence. If you have problems managing your emotions, seek professional assistance.

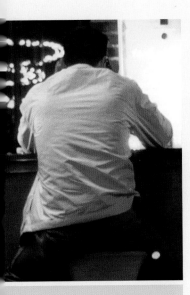

He didn't mean to

Often when people find themselves the victims of abuse, the tendency is either to blame themselves or to provide excuses for the abuser. If you are the victim of any kind of domestic abuse, remember the following:

• An unhappy childhood, stress, problems at work, or financial difficulties are not reasons for treating someone else badly.

• It's not your fault. You didn't ask for it, you didn't make him do it, and you didn't deserve it.

• Not talking about it won't make it go away. If you can't bring yourself to contact a support group, at least tell a friend who can help you take the next step.

• Retaliating will not help. Getting revenge on an abuser usually backfires. The best revenge is taking care of yourself.

• There's always a way out. Don't use financial obligations, the lease on your apartment, timing, or any other excuse for not breaking up with him, leaving, or taking action to get help for yourself.

• It won't get better. If you're telling yourself this, it's because you're afraid to end it. Get help and get away.

• Don't tell yourself that "it's not that bad." Any form of abuse is too much abuse, and there's no reason to tolerate it.

necessarily abuse either. They're not pleasant, but these things sometimes happen between people in a relationship.

Behavior becomes abuse when it's done deliberately to hurt or control someone. Trying to prevent a partner from going back to school, hanging out with friends, or changing jobs can be forms of abuse if your motivation in stopping him has more to do with what you fear his desires mean instead of what they really mean. Ridiculing a partner's ideas, appearance, or actions because it makes you feel good to put him down is abuse.

For a relationship to be healthy, both partners have to respect and support one another. Of course there are going to be fights and disagreements sometimes, but these situations can still be handled with love and respect. It's when one partner treats the other as if he's less worthy of respect that abuse occurs.

People abuse others for many reasons: to cover up their own feelings of powerlessness and inadequacy, because of addiction, or because of behaviors experienced or learned as children. But reasons are not excuses. If you find yourself involved with a partner who abuses you in any way, it is not your responsibility to help him or to make the situation better. It is your responsibility to get out of that relationship and, if necessary, seek protection or counseling to deal with it.

You, the abuser

If you are a person who is subjecting someone else to abusive behavior, it is important that you get help, either through a support group or a therapist. Similarly, if you recognize abusive behavior in someone else, encourage the men involved to seek help. No one benefits from keeping quiet about abusive situations.

Abusive behavior can also manifest itself in sexual behavior. Forcing a partner to engage in sexual activity he isn't comfortable with, just because you want to, is abusive. Subjecting him to humiliation or belittling his sexual abilities is

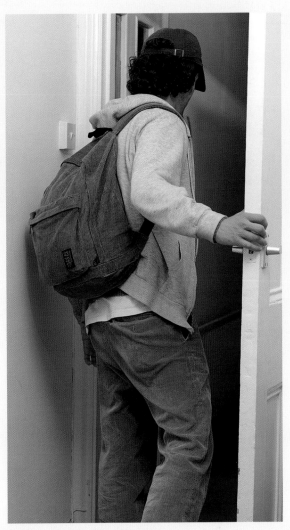

IF YOU FEEL that you are in any kind of danger from a partner's behavior, leave before the situation escalates and go somewhere safe.

also abuse (and to be clear, we're not talking about consensual S&M here). Cheating on a partner, and making sure he finds out, is another manifestation of abuse, as is leading someone on when you know you're not interested in them. Again, healthy sexual relationships, whether between partners or one-night stands, require that you respect your partners enough not to do anything to hurt them.

The erotic force of sex isn't diminished by remembering that your partners are people with feelings: Relationships are worthless if you don't respect the people in them and demand equal respect back. When we respect other people, we won't do anything to hurt them, and when we respect ourselves we won't let anyone hurt us.

Birthday blues?

Birthdays can be a big deal for some people, and not in a good way. Many of us cringe when we look at the calendar and see another Big Day coming around. We don't want the parties. We don't want a fuss. We just want to be left alone.

Well, get over it. Instead of hiding from your birthdays—particularly the ones that end in 5s and 0s—make them an occasion for big celebrations. Ignoring them isn't going to keep you from getting older, so you might as well give in and have fun. Even if you have to do it yourself, plan something.

You should also take some time on or around your birthday to reflect on the past year and look ahead to the next one. Birthdays, even more than the New Year, are excellent times for setting some goals for yourself. Don't try to overhaul your entire life, just pick a couple of things you might like to work on or a few things you want to achieve. See these through for a year and then when you reach your next Big Day you'll be ready to set a couple more goals for yourself.

Aging and age-related problems

Keeping fit and healthy as we grow older

Aging is one of those things we don't talk about very much as gay men. In fact, many of us actively fear growing older because we think it means losing our looks and not being the hot young things we once were (or at least thought we were). We call older men who dare to hang out at bars and clubs trolls, implying ugliness and desperation. We rarely see older gay men portrayed as sexual people and too often we relegate them to the roles of funny old queens, sugar daddies, or elder statesmen, whose primary function is to be witty but asexual. Well, it's high time to put this kind of backward thinking to bed and to celebrate the older man for what he is.

Age awareness

"How old are you?" It's not a question everyone likes to answer, but what constitutes "older" depends on your mindset. To guys in their early 20s, 30 may seem old, while to those who are well into their 30s, 40 and even 50 may still seem pretty young. It doesn't really matter where you think older begins; how you approach aging is the same whether you're hitting 25 or heading for the far side of 75.

The most important part of the aging process is accepting that our lives and our bodies change with the passing of time. As a result, the way we look at things, including sex and our relationships, changes, too. Acknowledging and working with these changes allows us to get the most out of our lives at every age, while doggedly attempting to hold back the hands of time will only result in frustration.

Acting your age

"Act your age" is one of those tricky pieces of advice. Just because you're, say, 55, doesn't mean you can't go out dancing, and just because you're 20 doesn't mean you *have* to go out dancing. But you might want to consider your age when you make certain decisions. We've all seen them (and some of us have been them): the guys trying way too hard to hold on to an image of themselves as being 23 forever.

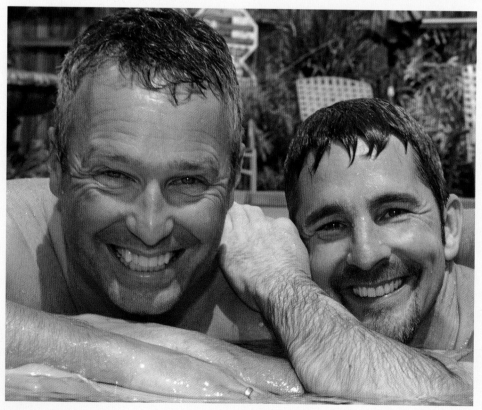

THINK ABOUT ALL THE THINGS that make you feel happy—there's no reason why you shouldn't enjoy them to the fullest, regardless of your age.

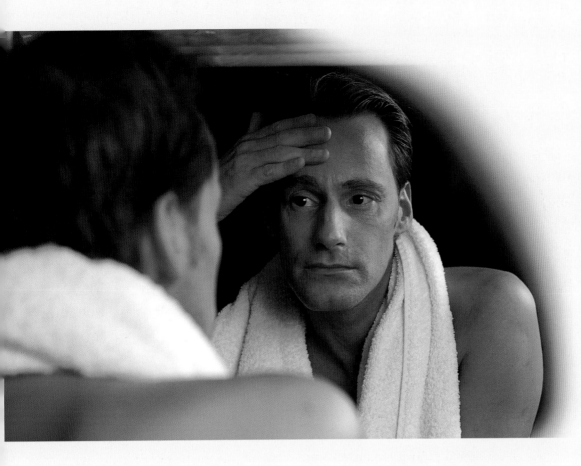

PHYSICAL AGING is quite natural. Value your body and remind yourself that what makes you desirable is the air of self-confidence, calm, and happiness that surrounds you.

Aging gracefully

Growing older doesn't mean fading away. The older we get, the more interesting we should become because we've been storing up experiences, making friends, and learning about who we are. Don't let those things go to waste. Use them to your advantage. Here are some hints:

• Don't let your sense of style get dusty. You don't have to keep up with the latest trends, but don't turn into your father or even your grandfather. Dress to look good.

• Share what you know. Consider volunteering or becoming a mentor, perhaps to a younger gay person. We all have a lot to offer those coming up after us.

• Maintain your friendships. As we age it's particularly nice to have a close group of friends to share experiences with. Don't neglect birthdays, anniversaries, and other special occasions.

• Don't live in the past. Sure, it's great to hold on to those special memories, but don't ever consider your best days behind you. You should always look forward.

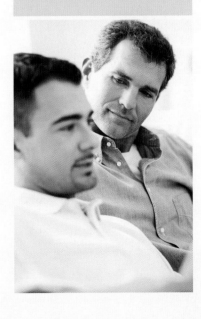

Determined not to let age get the best of them, they dress from the pages of Abercrombie & Fitch, spend hours in the gym and tanning salon, and insist on keeping up with the latest trends in music, fashion, and perhaps club drugs.

This kind of behavior is sad, sad, sad. I'm sure these fellows would say they're not letting age affect them, but what they're really doing is hanging on to a fantasy. Instead of figuring out who they are now, they're clinging to who they were 5, 10, 15, or 20 years ago. And when eventually they dissolve into a pile of bronzer, hair gel, and botox they'll do so wondering what became of their lives.

Compare this to the men who allow their lives to grow and change with every year, the men who cultivate a wide circle of intimate friends and a wide variety of interests. These men are seldom afraid of aging because they understand that although growing older means that things don't stay the same it doesn't mean that you can't undertake new adventures and learn to see things from new perspectives.

This includes changes in sexuality. As we age our bodies naturally change. Perhaps our physiques change, or we don't have as strong an interest in sex as we did earlier in our lives. Maybe we encounter difficulties with achieving erections or orgasm. These things happen, but usually there are ways in which we can try to counteract them.

The power of positive thinking

But the biggest defense against decreasing sexuality is the way we think about sex. If you expect every encounter to be the mind-blowing kind of sex you had when you were 20, you're probably going to be disappointed. Instead, if you learn to express sexuality in a variety of ways, you'll have a sex life that continues pretty much as long as you want it to. This means seeing the male body as something beautiful and erotic, not just when it's young and perfect, but in all its forms. It means thinking about yourself and about other men as sexual people at every different stage of life.

Media images of gay men don't help with this. Porn stars are, not surprisingly, young and buff. We don't often sexualize men with graying hair, a few extra pounds, and bad knees. And it's too bad because what older men might not have in the "perfect" body department they more than make up for in the experience department. More than that, they're generally more interesting people than their younger counterparts and that in itself can be incredibly erotic.

Aging successfully involves paying attention to both your physical and your emotional health. Physically, growing older brings many changes, and regular check-ups, eating correctly, and getting enough exercise are all-important components of maintaining your overall health.

The better you feel physically, the better your outlook on life will be, and this includes your attitudes toward sex.

Aging and your sex life

Eventually you are likely to encounter some physical challenges when it comes to sex. It's important to face these head-on and not ignore them. Too many men allow physical problems that are easily resolved to interfere with active sex lives, either because they consider the diminishing of their sexual lives to be expected or because confronting these issues is too embarrassing.

Aging-related issues can occur in any relationship, but may be more obvious or problematic in relationships involving partners

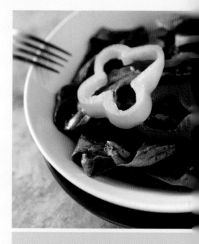

A SIGNIFICANT AGE difference between you and your partner may mean having to adjust to different levels of sexual interest as the relationship progresses.

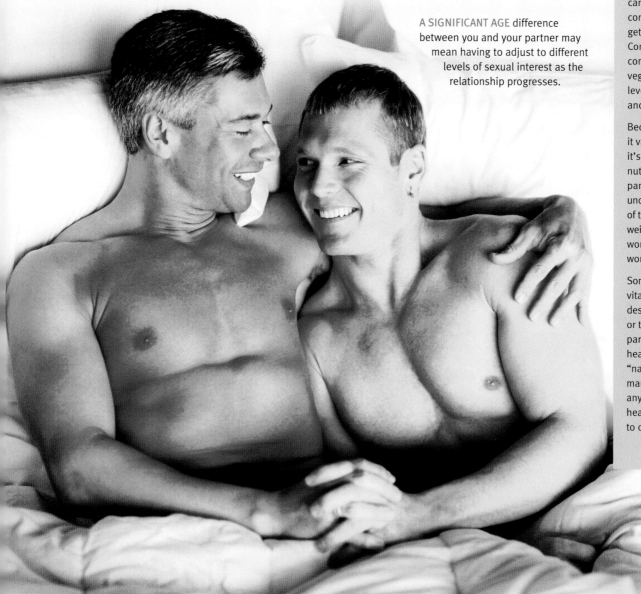

Food for thought

As we grow older it becomes increasingly important to watch our diet because what we eat often has an important effect on how we feel. Diets heavy in fats and sugars can make you feel tired, and may contribute to health problems that get in the way of sexual enjoyment. Conversely, diets rich in proteins, complex carbohydrates, and vegetables may increase energy levels, reduce excess weight, and promote overall health.

Because aging can bring with it various health conditions it's important to discuss your nutritional needs with your doctor, particularly if you're considering undertaking any type of diet. Many of these affect more than just your weight, so understanding how diets work and specifically how they work on *you* is important.

Some men may benefit from taking vitamins or other supplements designed to promote overall health, or to address health concerns particular to men (such as prostate health). There are more and more "natural" supplements being marketed—again, before taking anything that might affect your health, consult with a physician to determine if it's right for you.

of different ages. A 30-year-old man whose partner is in his 50s, for example, may (but not necessarily will) find that his lover isn't interested in being sexual as often as he is. If this occurs, it's important to discuss it, rather than ignoring the situation or allowing it to create additional issues.

As an individual, whether partnered or single, it is how you see yourself as you age that will have the most bearing on whether others find you sexually appealing and whether you enjoy an active sex life or not. A confident man creates an aura of sexiness, so learning to view yourself as an attractive, sexual person will help you create an impression that others find attractive as well.

It's also important to remember that no matter how confident you are, you're never going to be sexually appealing to everyone, and that's true of men at any age. If someone you're interested in doesn't return the interest, don't assume that it's because of your age. Sure, there are guys out there who will discount someone as a sexual or romantic partner simply because of how old he is, but usually the reasons for attraction are much more complex.

An eye for the younger guy

While we're on this subject, just as it's bothersome when younger men automatically reject older men, it's equally troubling to see older men who only pursue only younger men. It's certainly okay to be attracted to certain types, and if younger guys are your thing then that's fine. But if you remove older guys from your pool of possible partners you're missing out on some great opportunities.

I'll be honest, for some of us, learning to see older men as sexually exciting can take a bit of practice. If you've never considered an older man sexually before, give it a try, if not in real life then in your fantasy life. Pick an older man you find attractive. Imagine being sexual with him. Does it arouse you? Does it bother you?

Honestly explore your feelings around the experience. Try masturbating to such a fantasy and see what happens.

In fact, try it anyway. Most of us are sexually aroused by what we're told is sexy or by what we see portrayed in sexual situations. Learning to be turned on by things outside this limited pool of options isn't always something that comes easily, particularly if it means revising our ideas of what's appealing. If we've never seen older men portrayed sexually, or if we've never thought of them in a sexual way, it isn't something that we'll naturally do. By trying it, we can teach ourselves to look for and find out what's sexy about older men.

If you're already in the older category yourself (and I'll let you decide if you are or not) then practice seeing yourself as sexual. If you're partnered, be sure to spend time with your guy where you enjoy one another's bodies. Give each other massages and talk about what you find arousing about one another. Explore yourselves sexually together, even if you think you've done it all already. Odd as it sounds, it's easy to fall out of the habit of seeing your partner as a sexual person, and we all need reminding once in a while.

Would like to meet

If you're single, finding partners means what it means for any man—first creating the life you want and then looking for someone to share it with. As an older man you might not find the bars good places to look for partners, but there are many different social, recreational, and political groups that provide opportunities for men of any age to get together. And if you're simply looking for sexual partners, there are different options. Sex clubs and internet chat rooms are two possibilities, and if you're feeling particularly entrepreneurial, you might even want to start up a sex group specifically for older men (and their admirers, too, if you like) in your own area.

On the go

Exercise is important at any stage of life, but as we age it's even more important to remain active. This doesn't mean that on your 50th birthday you have to start training for a marathon; it means finding a level of activity that's appropriate for your age and your physical conditioning.

Staying active not only keeps you looking good, it enhances your enjoyment of sex by improving your overall health. Cardiovascular activity is particularly beneficial to men as we age, because it improves circulation. Finding an activity you like, whether it is running, walking, or swimming is also an excellent way to stay energized and in good spirits. Try to do one or more of these forms of exercise a couple times a week and you'll reap the reward.

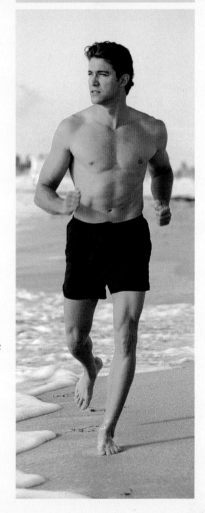

Further reading

NONFICTION BOOKS

The books that follow are excellent places to start reading about different aspects of gay sex, gay health, and gay life in general.

Alec Baldwin Doesn't Love Me
Michael Thomas Ford (Alyson Books)

Anal Pleasure and Health: A Guide for Men and Women
Jack Morin (Down There Press)

The Bear Handbook: A Comprehensive Guide for Those Who Are Husky, Hairy and Homosexual, and Those Who Love 'Em
edited by Ray Kampf (Harrington Park Press)

Bears on Bears: Interviews and Discussions
Ron Jackson Suresha (Alyson Books)

Boyfriend 101: A Gay Guy's Guide to Dating, Romance, and Finding True Love
Jim Sullivan (Villard)

Gay Sex: A Manual for Men Who Love Men
Jack Hart (Alyson Books)

Going Down: The Essential Guide to Oral Sex
Ben R. Rogers and Joel Perry
(Alyson Books)

The Ins and Outs of Gay Sex: A Medical Handbook for Men
Stephen E. Goldstone (Dell Publishing)

The Leatherman's Handbook and The Leatherman's Handbook II
Larry Townsend (LT Publications)

Male Erotic Massage: A Guide to Sex and Spirit
Kenneth Ray Stubbs, Ph.D. (Secret Garden)

Men Like Us: The GMHC Complete Guide to Gay Men's Sexual, Physical, and Emotional Well-Being
Daniel Wolfe (Ballantine Books)

OutSpoken: Role Models from the Lesbian and Gay Community
Michael Thomas Ford (Morrow)

Paths of Faith: Conversations about Faith and Spirituality
Michael Thomas Ford (Simon & Schuster)

100 Questions & Answers about AIDS: What You Need to Know Now
Michael Thomas Ford (Beech Tree Books)

Sex Adviser: The 100 Most Asked Questions about Sex Between Men
Tony Palermo (Alyson Books)

Sex, Orgasm, and the Mind of Clear Light: The Sixty-Four Acts of Gay Male Love
Jeffrey Hopkins (North Atlantic Books)

Sex Tips for Gay Guys
Dan Anderson (Griffin)

SM 101: A Realistic Introduction and Jay Wiseman's Erotic Bondage Handbook
Jay Wiseman (Greenery Press)

10 Smart Things Gay Men Can Do to Improve Their Lives
Joe Kort (Alyson Books)

The Soul Beneath the Skin: The Unseen Hearts and Habits of Gay Men
David Nimmons (Griffin)

Trust, the Hand Book: A Guide to the Sensual and Spiritual Art of Handballing
Bert Herrman (Alamo Square Press)

The Ultimate Guide to Anal Sex for Men
Bill Brent (Cleis Press)

Three the Hard Way: Tales of Three-Way Sex Between Men
edited by Austin Foxxe (Alyson Books)

The Voices of AIDS
Michael Thomas Ford (Morrow)

The World Out There: Becoming Part of the Lesbian and Gay Community
Michael Thomas Ford (The New Press)

FICTION

Reading erotic fiction can be an excellent way to turn yourself on or explore different aspects of sexual desire. These are some of the best on the market. As you'll see, most of them are published by Alyson Books, currently the leading publisher of gay erotica. Check out their website (www.alyson.com) for the latest offerings.

Bearotica:
Hot, Hairy, Heavy Fiction
edited by Ron Jackson Suresha
(Alyson Books)

Best Gay Erotica
edited by Rochard Labonte (Cleis Press)
Author's note: I was the first editor of this annual collection, which began in 1996. Each year's edition contains stories selected by a guest editor.

Cocksure
Bob Vickery (Alyson Books)

Dirty Words
M. Christian (Alyson Books)

Doing It for Daddy
edited by Pat Califia (Alyson Books)

Friction
edited by Jesse Grant (Alyson Books)
Author's note: This annual collection brings together the best fiction from some of the most popular erotic magazines.

Happily Ever After: Erotic Fairy Tales
for Men
edited by Michael Thomas Ford
(Masquerade Books)

Hard as They Come
Hal Reeves (Alyson Books)

Hardball
Tom T. Hitman (Alyson Books)

Hotter than Hell and Other Stories
Simon Sheppard (Alyson Books)

The Hounds of Hell and Other
SM Stories
Larry Townsend (LT Publications)

Jacked: The Best of Jack Fritscher
Jack Fritscher (Alyson Books)

Kinkorama
Simon Sheppard (Alyson Books)

Last Summer
Michael Thomas Ford (Kensington Books)

Looking for It
Michael Thomas Ford (Kensington Books)

Looking for Trouble
R.J. March (Alyson Books)

Masters of Midnight
Michael Thomas Ford et al
(Kensington Books)
Author's note: This collection of four novellas contains my story Sting.

Mr. Benson
by John Preston (Masquerade Books)

Muscle-Bound and Other Stories
Christopher Morgan (Alyson Books)

Roughed Up: More Tales of Gay Men,
Sex and Power
edited by Simon Sheppard and M. Christian

Tales from the Bear Cult
edited by Mark Henry (Palm Drive Publishing)

Tangled Sheets: The Erotica of
Michael Thomas Ford
Michael Thomas Ford
(Kensington Books)

Useful websites

The following listings are for groups, stores, and organizations that can be found online. Use them as a starting point for exploring the gay world and for gathering information on topics of interest to you.

BISEXUAL RESOURCES

Bi Men Network
www.bimen.org
An extensive collection of regional bisexual groups, both national and international. Provides advice, medical information, and the opportunity to network with over 100,000 members in a private forum.

BiNet USA
www.binetusa.org
A national umbrella network, providing links to various bisexual organizations and projects, and containing history and news on the bisexual community.

Bisexual Resource Center
www.biresource.org
Features many bisexual resources, particularly for those in the Boston area, as well as information on volunteering and otherwise encouraging bisexual pride.

EROTIC LITERATURE

A Different Light
www.adlbooks.com
Specializing in gay and lesbian literature, its extensive collection spans everything from education to fiction.

Alyson Books
www.alyson.com
Broad collection of LGBT products, ranging from comics and magazines to fictional and historical books.

Kensington Books
www.kensingtonbooks.com
Features gay and lesbian literature, as well as alternative romance novels.

GAY HEALTH ISSUES & SAFER SEX

LGBT Health Channel
www.gayhealthchannel.com
Developed and monitored by physicians, includes discussions on common health topics, and a forum in which more specific questions can be asked of doctors.

Gay & Lesbian Medical Association
www.glma.org
Provides news concerning health and public policy, in an effort to improve healthcare for the gay community.

Gay Men's Health Crisis
www.gmhc.org
Focuses on HIV/AIDS education, treatment, and prevention, and related political activity.

The Safer Sex Page
www.safersex.org
Essays and art exploring the gay identity in today's socio-political climate. Includes links to websites promoting safe sex.

The Sexual Health Network
www.sexualhealth.com
Provides information and discussions on STDs, sexual health, and sexual enjoyment.

GENDER RESOURCES

Gender.Org
www.gender.org
News and medical advisories relevant to transsexual and gender-variant people.

The International Foundation for Gender Education
www.ifge.org
Notices, events, and products concerning issues of transgenderism.

Intersex Society of North America
www.isna.org
Promotes understanding of the intersexual identity. Includes a medical advisory board.

GENERAL INTEREST

The Advocate
www.advocate.com
National news source covering gay and lesbian issues; it also features commentary on the arts, health, and cultural sensitivity.

Gay.Com
www.gay.com
News and health information, as well as travel, entertainment, business, and style.

National Association of Lesbian, Gay, Bisexual and Transgender Community Centers
www.lgbtcenters.org
Supports LGBT community centers, gives information to guide their development, and a directory of those established.

Planet Out
www.planetout.com
Guide to gay entertainment and
celebrity gossip, with comprehensive
personals section.

MENTAL HEALTH RESOURCES

Gay and Lesbian International Therapist Search Engine
www.glitse.com
GLITSE offers free and anonymous
services consisting of a national database
of referrals specific to the gay and lesbian
community. Search for a specialist online
who can help with gay and lesbian issues.

National Association of Lesbian & Gay Addiction Professionals
www.nalgap.org
Features resources aiming to educate,
prevent, and treat non-sexual addictions
affecting the LGBT community.

RESOURCES FOR OLDER GAY MEN

Apollo Network
www.apollonetwork.com
An informative site for older gay men
and those interested in them.

Gray Gay
www.graygay.com
News and advice for mature gay men
and their admirers.

Senior Action in a Gay Environment
www.sageusa.org
Social service agency for LGBT seniors that
details relevant activities and events.

RESOURCES FOR YOUNGER GAY MEN

The Coalition for Positive Sexuality
www.webcom.com/~cps
Covers important topics for teenagers,
including safe sex and attitudes towards gays.

OutProud
www.outproud.org
News, support, and encouraging literature
for and by queer youth.

Young Gay America
www.younggayamerica.com
Articles and advice on growing up gay
in modern America, including candid
sexual information.

Youth Resource
www.youthresource.com
Site devoted to education of young gay
and bisexual men; it features a peer
educator forum.

S&M

Gay Male S&M Activists
www.gmsma.org
Site devoted to raising awareness about
safe and responsible gay S&M.

Safer S&M Education Project
www.safersm.org
This website seeks to provide information
about safe S&M practices.

SEX SITES

Bad Puppy
www.badpuppy.com
Access newsgroups and art in addition
to video and images celebrating the
male physique.

Bedfellow
www.bedfellow.com
A seemingly endless collection of photo
and video images, featuring original
male models.

Cruising for Sex
www.cruisingforsex.com
Deemed one of the best websites
worldwide for "cruising," helping
gay men find one another.

SEX TOYS AND PRODUCTS

Blowfish
www.blowfish.com
Toys, books, videos, and other sex products
are all available from this website.

Good Vibrations
www.goodvibes.com
Resource for toys and other products.
Features *Good Vibes* magazine, and a museum
detailing the history of erotic novelties.

Grand Opening
www.grandopening.com
Award-winning site offering toys and
accessories for all, but featuring products
catered towards women in particular.

Glossary

Abuse
Deliberate behavior that causes ongoing or severe emotional or physical pain for another.

AIDS
Acquired Immune Deficiency Syndrome. Severe immunological disorder caused by the retrovirus HIV. It is transmitted primarily by exposure to infected body fluids, especially blood and semen.

Anal beads
Sex toy consisting of sphere-shaped beads strung together. When inserted or withdrawn from the anus they provide sexual pleasure.

Anal sex
Insertion of the penis, finger, tongue, or sex toy into the anus.

Anus
Opening to the rectum.

Bear
Hairy and often heavy man.

Bisexual
Capable of being erotically aroused by either men or women.

Blow job
Mouth-to-penis sex.

Bondage
Sexual play centered on control where one person wears restraints.

Butt plug
Dildo designed for insertion into the anus.

Cardiovascular
Having to do with the heart and blood vessels.

Casual sex
Sexual activity that does not involve an emotional component.

Chat room
Area on the internet where one can communicate in real time.

Circumcision
Removal of the foreskin around the glans.

Clone
Gay man of a standardized appearance. The proper "look" has changed over the decades.

Cock ring
Ring made of metal or leather placed around the penis and testicles to help sustain an erection.

Coming out
Acknowledgment and communication with family, friends, and acquaintances about your gay sexuality.

Condom
Latex sheath placed over the penis or sex toy during penetration. It can be used to decrease the risk of transmission of STDs.

Condyloma
Warty growth caused by the human papillomavirus (*see* HPV). It is usually benign, or non-cancerous.

Cruising
The playful art of seduction, sexual encounters, and erotic adventure.

Cruising grounds
Locations that are popular for the possibility of sexual encounters.

Cum *see* Semen

Date rape
Rape in which the person who commits the rape is known to the victim.

Depression
Chronic or recurrent mental state characterized by feelings of hopelessness, anxiety, loneliness, sadness, and lack of motivation and energy.

Dildo
Artificial penis usually made from rubber or silicone.

Doggie style
Anal sex with one partner behind the other.

Domestic violence
Physical, verbal, or emotional abuse that occurs in the home.

Drag queen
Man who dresses in women's clothes and affects women's mannerisms.

Ejaculation
Release of sperm and seminal fluid from the urethra during orgasm.

Enema
Introduction of a liquid into the colon through the anus for cleaning purposes.

Epididymis
Long, oval-shaped structure that stores sperm, at the upper rear of the testicle.

Erectile dysfunction
Inability to achieve and/or maintain an erection.

Erection
Rigid penis, due to spongy tissue of the penis engorging with blood.

Erogenous zone
Area of the body that, when physically stimulated, initiates or enhances sexual arousal.

Ex
Former lover.

Exhibitionism
Getting a thrill from engaging in sexual activity in front of a witness.

Fetish
Object to which someone attaches sexual desire.

Foreplay
Any activity that creates a sexy, romantic setting and mood.

Foreskin
Fold of skin over the glans.

Frottage
Rubbing the genitals against an object or partner. It can refer to sexual activity performed with the clothes on.

Fuck buddy
Casual sex partner, usually a friend or an acquaintance, with whom one has infrequent sex without total commitment.

G spot (male)
Erogenous zone activated by stimulating the prostate from within the anus.

"Gay cancer" *see* AIDS

Genital warts *see* HPV (human papillomavirus)

Giving head
Mouth-to-penis sex.

Glans
Head of the penis.

Gym bunny (Gym rat)
Gay man who affects a particularly fit body-type and way of dressing.

Hepatitis
Inflammation of the liver.

HIV-positive
Positive diagnosis for one of the strains of human immunodeficiency virus.

HPV (human papillomavirus)
Virus that causes genital warts. Over 70 types have been characterized. Unprotected contact with an infected person carries a 60 percent risk of infection.

Immune system
Body's natural defense against disruption caused by microbes and cancers.

Jerking/jacking off (JO)
Masturbation.

Kink
Behavior or activity that causes sexual fulfillment. It has the connotation of being eccentric or bizarre.

LGBT
Lesbian, gay, bisexual, or transgender. The term is used to describe the gay community as a whole.

Masochism
Deriving sexual gratification through receipt of pain or humiliation.

Masturbation
Self-stimulation of the genitals for erotic pleasure, often resulting in orgasm.

Missionary position
Anal sex with two partners facing each other.

Mummification
Wrapping a partner in plastic wrap.

Nipple clamp
Sex toy that clips or screws on, to provide pressure on the nipples.

Nonoxynol-9
Surface-acting spermicide commonly applied to condoms. It does not prevent transmission of HIV.

Orgasm
The climax of sexual excitement, which in men is accompanied by ejaculation.

Pelvic squeeze
An exercise that helps tighten the muscles around the anus.

Phone sex
Sexual play over the telephone, usually involving mutual masturbation.

Pornography
Writing, photography, film, art, spoken word, and computer-based media centered on sex.

Precum
Clear fluid released by the penis before ejaculation.

Prostate
Walnut-sized gland that surrounds the urethra. It secretes the seminal fluid discharged with sperm during ejaculation.

Rectum
The last segment of the large intestine, ending at the anus.

Rimming/rim job
Mouth-to-anus sex.

Sadism
Deriving sexual gratification through inflicting pain or humiliation on others.

S&M
Sadomasochism. Consensual sexual interaction between a dominant partner and a submissive partner. It centers on the taking, or giving up of, control.

Safer sex
Educated sex that uses techniques that limit the risk of transmitting or acquiring STDs.

"Safe word"
Password known between partners that will end S&M activity immediately.

Semen
Sperm and seminal fluid released during ejaculation.

Seminal fluid
Alkaline fluid secreted by the prostate gland and discharged with sperm during ejaculation.

Seminal vesicle
Folded, glandular structure in the testicle that is divided into sacs. Its secretion is one of the components of seminal fluid.

Sex club
Club where group sex is available.

Sex toys
Devices that are designed specifically for sexual pleasure.

Sphincter
Ring of muscle around the anus.

STDs
Sexually transmitted diseases. Diseases caused or propagated by sexual contact.

Steroids
Synthetic derivatives of the male hormone testosterone, used to add bulk to the body.

Testicle
Oval sex gland that is suspended in the scrotum and secretes sperm.

Testosterone
Naturally occurring male hormone. When administered as a drug it can cause gain in lean body mass, increased sex drive, and possibly aggressive behavior.

Three-ways
Sexual activity that includes three partners.

Transgender/transsexual
Person who has undergone or is preparing to undergo sex reassignment surgery.

Troll
A derogatory term for an unattractive older gay man.

Twink/Twinkie
Slang for a young gay man who is admired for his good looks and slim build, but not for his intellect.

Urethra
Canal leading from the bladder, discharging urine externally from the tip of the penis.

Urinary tract infection (UTI)
Bacterial infection of the urinary tract. It can also involve the kidney, bladder, and urethra.

Vanilla sex
Conventional sex, with the connotation of being boring.

Vas deferens
Secretory duct of the testicle.

Index

Picture credits

12: Alamy Images/Gianni Muratore (bl)
13: Corbis/PBNJ Productions (br)
14: Powerstock/ Orangestock (tr); Stockbyte (b)
15: Alamy Images/Directphoto.org (tc); Corbis/Randy Faris (br)
16: Kobal Collection/UnitedArtists/ Sebastian Lorey (tl)
17: Getty Images/Frank Micelotta (t); Powerstock/Superstock/Mitchel Gray (br)
18: Getty Images/Thinkstock (cl)
24: Photo Courtesy of Men Magazine © Speciality Publications 2003
30: Powerstock/Superstock/ Adamsmith (bl)

35: Stockbyte
37: Stockbyte
38: Masterfile UK/Kathleen Finlay (b); Queerstock (tr)
39: Alamy Images/ Bob Jones Photography (br); Queerstock (tc)
47: Alamy Images/David Hoffman
48-49: Alamy Images/ Bob Jones Photography (bl)
49: Magnum/Peter Marlow (tr)
52-53: Getty Images/Naile Goelbasi
53: Getty Images/Digital Vision/ Jack Slomovits (br)
54: Stockbyte (tr), (bl)
55: Masterfile UK/Dazzo
56: Getty Images/Philip Lee Harvey (bl)
57: Stockbyte
58: Stockbyte (tl); Getty Images/ Tipp Howell (bl)
59: Alamy Images/Directphoto.org (cr); Queerstock (tl)
61: Stockbyte
64: Stockbyte
65: Stockbyte (tr)
66: Zefa Picture Library/R. Elstermann (bl)
68: Stockbyte
70: Stockbyte (cl)
71: Stockbyte
72: Getty Images/Joe Schmelzer

74: Getty Images/Adri Berger (bl)
76: Getty Images/Photodisc Green/ Doug Menuez (tl); Getty Images/ Romilly Lockyer (bl)
80: Stockbyte
85: Stockbyte
103: Stockbyte
142: Corbis/Scott Houston (tl)
146: Queerstock (tl)
153: Getty Images/Photodisc/Tim Hall (tl)
154: Corbis/Sion Touhig
160: Getty Images/Photodisc/ Doug Menuez
164: Getty Images/Romilly Lockyer (b)
170: Getty Images/Hans Gelderblom (bc)
172-173: Getty Images/Dale Durfee
174: Stockbyte (br)
177: Retna Pictures Ltd/New Eyes (tl)
178: Queerstock; 179: Stockbyte (br)
180: Stockbyte (bl).

All other images © DK Images.
For further information see:
www.dkimages.com

Acknowledgments

Michael Thomas Ford would like to thank Daniel Cullinane for the introduction, Mitchell Waters for the good advice, and Jennifer Williams, Susan St. Louis, Sharon Lucas, Tina Vaughan, and Chuck Lang for everything else.

DK Publishing would like to thank Corinne Roberts and Lynne Brown for their tireless support; and Miesha Tate for jacket design.

Studio Cactus would like to thank all the models who appear in the book for their enthusiasm, professionalism, and, most of all, their sense of humor; Cloudbase Productions, The Perch, The Lemon Tree, and The Studio for location hire; Uwe at MASTERU/Leatherbound online shop (www.masteru.com) for the use of his props; Carnival Store for costume hire (www.carnivalstore.co.uk); She 'n' Me fetish shop (www.she-n-me.com); photographer Justin Slide and his assistants; makeup artists Anna Haig, Lisa Stokes, and Samantha Williams; Adam Moore for DTP work; Sue Gordon for editorial assistance; Zeb Korycinska for indexing; Alison Shakspeare for proofreading; and Emily Hawkins for model research.